COMMONSENSE BREASTFEEDING

A Practical Guide to the Pleasures, Problems, and Solutions

DIANE M. REUKAUF and

MARY ANNE TRAUSE, Ph.D.

With an introduction by
JOHN H. KENNELL, M.D. and
MARSHALL H. KLAUS, M.D.

ATHENEUM   NEW YORK   1988

Atheneum
Macmillan Publishing Company
866 Third Avenue, New York, N.Y. 10022
Collier Macmillan Canada, Inc.

Library of Congress Cataloging-in-Publication Data

Reukauf, Diane M.
    Commonsense breastfeeding.
    1. Breast feeding. I. Trause, Mary Anne. II. Title.
RJ216.R38   1987   649'.33   87–17503
ISBN 0–689–11761–2
ISBN 0–689–11867–8 (pbk.)

Macmillan books are available at special discounts for bulk
purchases for sales promotions, premiums, fund-raising, or
educational use. For details, contact:

Special Sales Director
Macmillan Publishing Company
866 Third Avenue
New York, N.Y. 10022

10 9 8 7 6 5 4 3 2 1

Printed in the United States of America

TO BETH, KATHRYN, AND MICHAEL,
who introduced me to motherhood and
other adventures,

AND TO BILL,
whose strength and good humor have
made this a happy journey.
D. M. R.

TO AMANDA AND TOMMY,
who continue to show me new pleasures
of motherhood,

AND TO PAUL,
who has doubled the pleasure by
sharing it all.
M. A. T.

Contents

Acknowledgments

MANY PEOPLE have played a part in the conception, shaping, and writing of this book. Those women we interviewed who shared their concerns and insights with us provided an abundance of information. We are grateful to them for their openness and generosity. The details of their experiences as breastfeeding mothers both directed and tested our thinking.

We find that our approach to families and their nursing infants has been profoundly influenced by John Kennell, Marshall Klaus, Sheila Kitzinger, and Betsy Lozoff. Their research, clinical work, and writings have introduced both professionals and the general public to some key issues of family development. They are all teachers in the fullest sense of the word. They continue to ask crucial questions; they have a passion to communicate what they know; and they do it well. Their understanding of the richness of parent-child relationships helped to guide our work.

We have benefited from the practical experiences of several professionals. JoAnne Scott, a certified lactation consultant, has worked with hundreds of women. Her contributions to this book reflect her sensitivity and her down-to-earth approach. We thank Meredith Wade of La Leche League International and Joyce Daniel and Bryn Burke, certified nurse midwives. We are fortunate to have these women as neighbors and friends who were interested in our project and who were willing to answer our questions as we progressed through the issues.

We also are grateful to the following people: Those La Leche League leaders and ASPO/Lamaze childbirth educators who expressed interest in this work, and who often introduced us to new breastfeeding mothers; the medical and nursing staffs in the neonatal unit and the librarians at Fairfax Hospital; our friends and colleagues from the Alliance for Perinatal Research and Services, Inc.; Lynn Moen of the Birth and Life Bookstore in Seattle; Karen Mendenhall, who worked with us in the early stages of this project; and Vonnie Malek and Lee Henderson, who did the bulk of our typing.

We are grateful for the assistance we received from Lynn Seligman, our agent, who liked the manuscript in the first place, and who has guided us through many stages of the work since then. We thank Susan Ginsberg, our editor at Atheneum, for her many valuable recommendations. Her questions challenged our thinking and led us to articulate more clearly our philosophy regarding the role of breastfeeding in women's lives.

We are thankful for the support we received from our families: our parents, Anne and Jim McVittie, and Rena and Jim Staigers, who gave us our first lessons in parenting, and who have always been enthusiastic about our endeavors; Hazel Reukauf and Sid Trause, whose attention and affection enrich our families' lives; our sisters, Rosemary Chidester, Joanie Staigers-Smith, and Jackie Staigers, who often were a source of good breastfeeding and mothering stories, and who always were a source of encouragement; and our husbands and children, who tolerated, in good humor, the many inconveniences created by moms who are writing a book.

Finally, we are enormously grateful to our friend Nikki Hardin. Nikki was the first person in the publishing business to show an interest in our ideas. She encouraged us to pursue the project, and she taught us to be comfortable with our own voices in the manuscript. Her sense of the written language and her sense of humor are powerful gifts she shared with us. We were fortunate to begin our work under her direction. In a very real sense, she is responsible for our ideas becoming a book.

Preface

THIS BOOK does not tell the whole truth about breastfeeding. It does tell the truth as it has been experienced by many women at different stages in the breastfeeding cycle. We interviewed over one hundred women who were beginning to breastfeed, or who were nursing their babies in the midst of active lives, or who were contemplating and carrying out the weaning process.

Because these women were mostly middle-class, urban and suburban mothers, the picture we present in this book may not accurately describe some of the circumstances of breastfeeding as they are experienced by a broader spectrum of contemporary women. A cross-cultural perspective probably would demonstrate many similarities, but also might reveal some interesting differences.

At times you may notice that we switch from "we" to "I" in presenting information. This is done when the material reflects the personal experiences of only one of us.

There is another pronoun issue we should acknowledge. We debated how to equally represent both genders in our references to babies (the old "he/she" dilemma). In the end, we felt confined by the current limitations of the English language. Therefore, we have chosen, *not* by reason of political or sociological considerations, to revert to the traditional use of "he" and "him" as pronouns that cover both sexes. This decision was based on our desire for clarity and simplicity. Since women's stories play such a large part in this book, the pronouns "she" and "her" appear frequently. It seemed convenient and less confusing to use "he" and "him" when referring to the baby.

In telling the stories in this book, we chose not to use the real names of the families we interviewed.

Introduction

John H. Kennell, M.D.
Marshall H. Klaus, M.D.

THIS IS a special book. Many mothers with breastfeeding experience—and those who have sought advice from other sources—will be amazed and delighted when they find that this book is so informative. So practical. So helpful. So easy to read. The suggestions are presented in such an easy style that you can imagine you are chatting with the authors in your living room.

The authors have a strong belief in the value of breastfeeding. Using anecdotes and advice from their own rich experience and from other women who have breastfed, they illustrate how to make breastfeeding a workable and enjoyable experience in our present-day situation—where women work, where there are heavy demands and schedules to meet. They explain how it is possible to start breastfeeding successfully, even in hospitals that are controlled by complex and, in some cases, rigid practices. The authors know their subject well and they have woven together the known facts as well as many unique observations that have only recently been made.

The biology of milk production probably evolved over thousands of centuries. The physiology and the behaviors associated with breastfeeding appear to have resulted from an adaptation of human biology to the life of hunting and gathering lived by our early predecessors. They carried their babies on their bodies for the first two to four years of life, breastfed for short periods thirty to forty times in a twenty-four-hour period, and walked 1,500 miles a year to forage and hunt for food.

The authors describe the complexities of feeding behavior between the mother and her infant in a thoughtful fashion. They show unusual sensitivity in understanding that a mother requires much more than just a list of do's and don'ts. They appreciate that a mother needs information presented in a way that fosters belief in herself. Donald Winnicott was well aware of this when he wrote: "The mother is probably the one person who can introduce the world to the baby in a way that makes sense to the baby. She knows how to do this, not through any training and not through being clever, but just because she's the natural mother. Mother's milk does not flow like an excretion; it is a response to a stimulus—a stimulus of the sight, the smell and the feel of her baby and the sound of the baby's cry that indicates need."(Donald W. Winnicott, p.111).

The authors neatly describe the multitude of interlocking and reciprocal interactions that occur as the mother is breastfeeding. As they have noted, these behaviors do not occur in a chainlike sequence, but each behavior triggers many others. Thus, the effect of the interaction is more like that of a stone dropping into a pool, causing a multitude of ever-increasing rings, rather than that of a chain, where each link leads to another. To the infant the mother gives her touch, eye-to-eye contact, warmth, and especially her love. She sets the time and the rhythm, and of course provides the unique nutritional and immunologic characteristics of the milk as well as the antibodies that protect the infant from infection. The baby, on its part, stimulates the mother's oxytocin and prolactin, moves in rhythm, and in a sense answers, as the mother speaks.

Although much has been written about various behavioral aspects of breastfeeding, little has been said, in our own society, about the relaxing and almost psychotropic effect that the mother senses during and following feeding. We do not believe that this relaxing and soothing effect occurs by chance. It probably helps to bring the mother and baby together, creating the unique tie that becomes stronger with each feeding and permits mother and infant to be linked in a symbiotic union.

The authors of *Commonsense Breastfeeding* have a full knowledge of the basic biology of breastfeeding. They have adapted the physiologic principles to fit with present-day practices in today's drastically different world for women. They approach breastfeeding by helping each woman evaluate and consider what would be best for her own family situation. We are especially fortunate that the authors have produced a thoughtful, sensitive, and appropriate book for the modern-day family.

✿1✿

Reflections on Breastfeeding

✿

*I must say it's a bit of
an adjustment. Give it time.*

—A NEW MOTHER

PREGNANCY. Childbirth. Breastfeeding. All are parts of
the same cycle. And at each point in the cycle there are facts we need
to know, changes we want to understand, and emotions we try to
handle. When I attended those first childbirth classes with my husband, I did so with the intention of becoming informed. The ratio-
nale went something like this: If I know and understand more of
what I might expect, then I will be less surprised as labor and
delivery progress; if I am less surprised, then I will be less disturbed
and frightened. What actually happened went something like this:
Each week I heard more information that surprised and disturbed
me. (Labor could be *how* long? How many people would be watching my "bulging perineum" as I pushed? They had to be kidding
about "passing urine" right there on the labor bed!) I spent a good
deal of time imagining that for *me* things would be very different
(very short, very private, and very clean).

In the end, of course, most of us benefit from such educational
and emotional preparation. What is perhaps unfortunate is that,

when it's our turn, we get prepared all at once. Whether it's for childbirth or breastfeeding, preparation in our culture today is apt to happen all of a sudden. And some of the things we all-of-a-sudden learn about breastfeeding can be confusing or discouraging. (It can take *how* long to complete a feeding? Sore nipples? I might leak?) Once again, I can find myself thinking that it will probably be very different for me (very short, very comfortable, very clean). As one mother remarked, "I was surprised that breastfeeding was such hard work in the beginning. I had read about how convenient it was."

Although there are some basic facts and techniques about the mechanics of breastfeeding, women fashion a broad range of nursing styles for themselves and their babies. We interviewed women who breastfed for three weeks, three months, a year, or more. Of women who worked outside the home, some stopped nursing when they returned to work. Others chose to continue nursing either by leaving formula for their babies or by providing their own breastmilk, which they pumped or expressed. Even women who were not employed outside their homes followed a variety of breastfeeding methods and styles.

Individual mothers need to make individual decisions. There is considerable pressure on women to succeed, to do it all, to do it right. We set goals and believe that, with determination, we can accomplish anything. Sometimes having orgasms, giving birth naturally, and breastfeeding are seen in the same terms: feats to be accomplished, ways to improve our sense of competence. We focus on how well we can perform. This pressure can make human experiences like making love and breastfeeding much more difficult.

In addition, although the world we live in intellectually supports breastfeeding, it doesn't support it in a practical sense. Mothers today tend to be on the go, with many commitments outside the home. Restaurants, stores, and workplaces don't invite, approve, or often even allow breastfeeding. Throughout history, women have contributed to the livelihood of their families. Today, however, many of their activities take them physically away from their homes and children.

The world we live in is not necessarily compatible with the

realities of breastfeeding. As a result, many women choose not to breastfeed. Fortunately, formulas have been developed that allow babies to thrive without mother's milk. Nevertheless, there has been a resurgence in breastfeeding. The challenge for women who want to breastfeed is how to manage in light of the demands imposed on women today by society and by women themselves.

Our intention in this book is to reduce the pressure and provide information and support for mothers who want to breastfeed, for as long as they choose. Depending on the changing facts and circumstances of your life, you will create a breastfeeding experience that works for you and your family. We met women who decided to stop breastfeeding earlier than they had originally planned. We also spoke to mothers who were surprised that they continued to nurse longer than they had envisioned.

Generally, we like to think of breastfeeding as a perfectly natural activity and process. Some aspects of it, however, do not come naturally. Most of us have had little or no experience with breastfeeding before we begin the process ourselves. It is likely that we grew up without observing breastfeeding or overhearing conversations about this mother-infant activity. In a sense, we've been deprived of a wide variety of collective memories: the newborn who wouldn't nurse for days, the aunt who was ill but continued to breastfeed her child, the twelve-month-old who still refused solids.

But even if you have had limited exposure to the experience of breastfeeding, you may have sources of information. Perhaps you have friends or relatives who nursed their babies. You may have observed them closely. Perhaps you have read about breastfeeding. At the very least, you know that women have breastfed their babies since the beginning of time, and, understanding the basics, you simply intend to let nature take its course. Thus you may begin your own experience with breastfeeding assuming that, as a standard woman with a standard baby, you will proceed with nursing more or less instinctively. There are only three problems with this line of thinking: (1) the idea that nursing is instinctive; (2) the idea that you're a standard woman, and (3) the idea that you've given birth to a standard baby.

First, we have learned that among primates, including humans, nursing is *not* entirely instinctive. Derrick and Patrice Jelliffe in their book *Human Milk in the Modern World* explain that the breastfeeding process is partly learned behavior; females gain information from other females, mainly by observation and example. The authors tell of the first two chimpanzees born in a zoo in 1920. They were born to a nonwild mother, a female chimp who had never seen baby chimps suckle. As a result, she did not nurse her own babies and they died. In 1974 a nonwild female gorilla was "taught" about breastfeeding. During her pregnancy, she was shown films of nursing gorillas. She went on to nurse her offspring successfully.

Second, although you may be a standard woman in the sense of being "normal," there may be many things about you that make you different from the other nursing mothers you've known or read about. Perhaps you are returning to work soon, or your husband is less than enthusiastic about your nursing. Maybe you crave more order in your life than nursing seems to allow or you have sensitive skin and worry that there'll be no end to nipple soreness.

Finally, what about that standard baby of yours? If your baby is full term and healthy, he comes with three valuable reflexes that make nursing possible. He can root (turn his head toward anything that touches his cheek), he can suck, and he can swallow (see Chapter 2). If your baby was born more than six weeks early, he may need some time to mature before he can coordinate sucking and swallowing. Eventually he will (see Chapter 4). Nonetheless, even though your baby may have the necessary "standard" equipment to become a real pro at nursing, he may exhibit a style of nursing that surprises, confuses, or disturbs you. His style may not match either your picture of the typical nursing baby or your recollection of other nursing babies. A newborn comes to you with his own temperament, which can affect his style of nursing. Some babies latch on well and nurse efficiently right from the beginning, but others take days to get used to the idea. Still others may nurse only a little at a time, then rest a while, then nurse again. One style is not better than another for your developing infant, although *you* may have a preference.

The popular notions about breastfeeding, including the idea

that it is a convenient, effortless, and instinctive way to feed a baby, can cause some trouble for a new mother. If you haven't questioned some of these notions beforehand, you may be dismayed by your feelings of ineptitude when you put your baby to your breast for the first time. Often the first "feeding" results in several attempts with little actual nursing. Countless mothers and infants who begin this way go on to develop easy and gratifying nursing relationships. If you expect some early temporary difficulties, you will be better prepared for the reality of beginning breastfeeding.

Since breastfeeding is not entirely instinctive, you will need some facts as you begin your own nursing experience. Many of these facts will be provided in the following chapters. Since there is great variety among mothers and infants, you might benefit from learning about the behaviors and styles of other women and their babies. We have interviewed mothers who were in various stages of the breastfeeding cycle, from childbirth to weaning. We saw how breastfeeding influences and is influenced by their lives. In the chapters that follow, we describe breastfeeding mothers—their problems and pleasures, their dilemmas and decisions. We hope this combination of factual information and personal experiences will help you as you progress through your own breastfeeding experience.

As we begin, we think it is important to explain the principles that have provided the framework for our discussions. Our responses to nursing problems and our treatment of breastfeeding issues are influenced by the following concepts:

- The newborn is a capable and sensitive person.
- Breastmilk is the preferred food for a baby.
- Breastfeeding is meant to be unrestricted.
- Women tend to feel ambivalent about breastfeeding.

A Newborn Is a Capable and Sensitive Person

In childbirth classes, parents-to-be are often interested in the particular capabilities of a newborn. "When can they see?" "Will the baby be able to tell the difference between me and my wife?" "Aren't the first smiles just gas?" These questions indicate something beyond curiosity. Parents want to know what matters to a baby. If nothing matters, if nothing registers in the baby's brain for the first several weeks, then the way the parent behaves toward the baby cannot make much difference. On the other hand, what if the infant is actually paying attention and processing much of what is happening to him and around him?

Research confirms what most parents of newborns suspect. The new baby *is* sensitive to his environment. The evidence tells us that the way we hold a baby, feed him, speak and sing to him, entertain and respond to him *does* make a difference in the baby's response. He is not simply a cuddly or unpredictable bundle waiting to turn into something real at three or six months. A newborn is capable of seeing, hearing, smelling, and experiencing pain and pleasure.

The newborn can see. As soon as he is born, he is able to focus his eyes. He sees best at a distance of seven to ten inches. Newborns also show visual preferences. They spend more time looking at and following a human face than they do looking at an inanimate object.

The newborn can hear. He is more responsive to the soft, higher pitch of female voices. Dr. T. Berry Brazelton suggests that many of us demonstrate an understanding and acceptance of the infant's hearing pattern in the way we verbally communicate to an infant. Men and women and even children will soften their voices and use a higher pitch when they talk to babies.

The newborn can smell. After the fifth day of life, he can discriminate his own mother's odor from that of other mothers. The infant, when given the choice of two breast pads, will selectively turn toward his own mother's.

The newborn experiences pleasure. A one-week-old infant will smile fleetingly, not from gas but because his tummy is satisfied or because he hears soft sounds. By one month the smiles begin to be more frequent and are more likely to be related to people. The cry of the newborn, often caused by hunger, cold, interrupted sleep or feedings, being dressed or undressed, or being left alone, is powerful evidence that a newborn is capable of experiencing displeasure, frustration, and pain.

Whether you are living with a "good" baby, who places few demands on you, or an active baby, who seems to need you all the time, it is important to see your newborn as someone who *does* notice the world around him—the smells, the noises, the activity, the touches. It is clear that he will need help from you to get relief from pain (hunger, thirst, cold, tummyaches, and the like). In addition, he may frequently need help handling his periods of frustration or boredom. (In that way, a baby is not so different from most grown-ups.) Also, a baby usually needs your assistance to help him experience delight or pleasure. As the research tells us, and as most parents suspect, the newborn is not on his way to becoming a person. At birth he is already a fairly capable individual.

If we thought our newborns couldn't hear our voices, didn't see our faces, and didn't experience pleasure and pain, we might approach feeding them very differently. But observations make it clear that the satisfying feeding experience is based on a relationship between two sensitive, responsive persons. Breastfeeding is not strictly a physiological act to be performed efficiently. It emerges from a relationship that recognizes and respects the individuality of each partner.

Breastmilk Is the Preferred Food for a Baby

A few years ago it was popularly believed that it didn't matter whether a baby was breastfed or bottle-fed as long as he was fed lovingly. We now understand that this statement is not accurate in regard to the infant's physical health. Breastfed babies tend to be healthier. Human milk is widely accepted as the perfect food for babies. It can fulfill all the infant's nutritional needs for at least the first six months of life.

Dr. Ruth Levy Guyer, an immunologist and a writer, explains that more than one hundred ingredients have already been identified in mother's milk and there are probably others which available scientific methods cannot measure.

Formula manufacturers contend that they have "humanized" cow's milk with supplements so that commercial infant formulas are essentially the same as and as good as mother's milk. But it is impossible to manufacture a perfect formula: all of the beneficial ingredients in human milk are not known, many of them cannot be made outside the body and many cannot withstand the types of processing which would be involved in putting them into formulas. The many ways in which infants profit from breastfeeding are not fully understood, but medical studies clearly show that nursing gives newborns an enormous health advantage over bottle-fed infants—an advantage that persists throughout life (Guyer and Freivogel, p. 2).

The following list is drawn from facts scientists know about human milk and should give you an idea of its special suitability for babies.

• Colostrum, the yellowish substance first secreted by the breasts, has been called an antibody cocktail because it is so rich in bacteria-fighting substances. The newborn who gets colostrum is given a "shot" of antibodies to help protect him from infection as he adjusts to life outside his mother's bacteria-free uterus. One study has shown that the infection rate of premature and sick infants was substantially decreased by giving them just three teaspoons of colostrum each day.

• Some ingredients of mother's milk, once it has come in, can help protect the baby from infection. Since an infant's immunological system does not fully develop for about two years, the immunities that your breastmilk provides are crucial. Some ingredients promote the growth of beneficial bacteria in the baby's intestines. These "good" or "friendly" bacteria help the infant digest his food and help to "crowd out" other, potentially harmful bacteria. With all this protection, the breastfed baby is likely to have fewer infections. In addition, when the mother is exposed to diseases, her own body will attempt to fight them off by producing antibodies. The antibodies she produces are passed to her baby through the milk and further protect him against specific diseases.

• Breastfed babies have fewer allergies. Foreign proteins (as found in cow's milk or soy-based formulas) are among the chief causes of allergies in children. The baby's immature digestive system is not able to process this foreign material. As a result, the inappropriate protein stays in the intestines or passes through the immature, permeable intestinal wall, where it sensitizes the baby's immune system. It seems that it is this very early sensitization that leads to allergies later in life. If the baby has no cow's milk products until his intestines are more mature and less permeable (at least six months of age), there is less chance of developing allergies.

• Human milk is easy for babies to digest. Cow's milk is high in protein, but it is not the right kind for babies. It tends to form a hard, bulky, indigestible curd in the baby's stomach. Mother's milk is lower in protein, but the protein it contains is more easily and more entirely used by the baby's body. It forms a soft curd, which is readily disgested and leaves the stomach more quickly.

• Mother's milk is high in cholesterol, a component which is important in brain development. Current research indicates that if your baby's body learns to metabolize cholesterol in the beginning of life, he may have fewer problems with it as an adult.

• The composition of a mother's milk alters as her baby grows. The quantities of some nutrients increase, others decrease. The milk seems to change to meet the changing needs of the maturing baby. It is for this reason that mothers of premature infants receive so much encouragement to provide their *own* milk for their babies (in addition to whatever milk is available through milk banks). Their milk is composed of ingredients in the proportions specifically needed by their premature infants. Most manufactured formulas are standard, providing the same food for the one-day-old as for the nine-month-old, even though these babies' needs are very different.

Breastfeeding Is Meant to Be Unrestricted

Once upon a time there was only breastfeeding. When a baby indicated a need to nurse, the mother offered her breast. No one checked a clock. Much later in time, when sterilized bottles and rubber nipples became available, there was formula-feeding. The growing respect for science led to babies receiving measured feedings at measured intervals. At the present time, women are returning to breastfeeding in ever-increasing numbers. But there's a hitch. Today a woman may choose breastfeeding but may be encouraged to apply the principles of bottle-feeding. Thus she attempts to restrict the number of feedings in each twenty-four-hour period, and she attempts to restrict the amount of time the baby nurses at each feeding. This restricted breastfeeding doesn't work—or it works poorly—for three reasons. *First, limiting breast-feeding will limit your milk supply.* Your baby's frequent periods of sucking encourage your body to make milk. *Second, mother's milk contains different ingredients than formula.* The ingredients in breast-milk are digested easily and more quickly, and therefore a breastfed baby is likely to feel hunger well before a formula-fed baby does. *And finally, nursing is more than a process of getting a certain amount of food into your baby.* It is also a way to calm and comfort babies. Thus, even if your baby is not ravenous, he may sometimes need to nurse for the security and soothing effect it offers him. (This has been referred to as nonnutritional nursing.)

Understanding the diversity in approaches to breastfeeding—restricted versus unrestricted—helps explain why nursing may work for some women and not for others. Reports such as "I tried to breastfeed our first baby, but I never seemed to have enough milk," often come from mothers who were advised to restrict their nursing (four minutes each side; only every four hours). In our discussions of breastfeeding in this book, we begin with the premise that establishing a good milk supply and a relaxed, positive nursing relationship with your baby is difficult—if not impossible—when breastfeeding is seriously restricted and when it is based on principles intended for formula-feeding.

It seems that among animals who nurse their young there are two basic styles of infant care. Among some land mammals there is considerable contact between mother and baby. The infant may be carried by the mother, or he may follow her closely. Nursings take place every one to two hours or even more frequently. This group is called the constant-contact or continuous-contact species.

In the second group of mammals, there is considerably less mother-infant contact. The baby is tucked away in a safe place (a nest or burrow), and the mother goes off for extended periods of time. Nursings may take place every two to fifteen hours. Such mammals constitute the intermittent-contact species.

There is another difference between these two groups. Their milk is different. Each group produces milk that seems especially suited to the way its mothers care for their infants. Thus, the baby deer who receives a feeding only twice a day is provided with milk that is rich in protein and fat. He survives and thrives feeding only once every twelve hours. The baby chimpanzee, who follows his mother and rides on her back and feeds frequently, is drinking a milk which has a low concentration of protein and fat. This kind of milk needs to be ingested frequently (Lozoff and Brittenham, pp. 480–83).

Where do *you* fit in? Human milk has been tested. The concentrations of protein and fat have been measured. Welcome to the constant-contact species! The composition of your milk, with low concentrations of protein and fat, most resembles the milk of animals who nurse frequently, almost continuously. The kind of milk you make is needed often by your newborn.

This is not to say that all human infants will nurse continuously (although some days it may *seem* that way), but it does help to explain many things about human babies. With this information in mind, it might be easier to understand why it's so difficult to get most babies on a schedule, why some babies seem to be feeding all the time, and why many babies don't sleep through the night.

Being a member of a constant-contact species may not be your first choice. It may not be compatible with your lifestyle, your temperament, or your career aspirations. There may be times when you'll wish you were like the deer, feeding your baby twice a day, with plenty of time off in between for personal endeavors, like foraging in the woods for nuts and berries. Nonetheless, it is important to understand the nature of your milk and the style of infant care it suggests.

It has been only very recently in the history of the human species that mothers have begun to restrict infant feedings and tuck their babies away in safe places (cribs, playpens, wind-up swings, day-care centers). The style of infant care that included carrying the baby and providing frequent feedings—a style that persisted for more than one million years—is no longer prevalent (except in nonindustrialized societies). Women's lives—mothers' lives—may have changed dramatically in the last two hundred years, but the composition of human milk remains the same.

This information may seem to suggest that breastfeeding is incompatible with the lives of most women today. It's difficult to imagine a woman who would be free constantly to carry and nurse her baby. Nor is that necessary. You will read, in later chapters, about nursing mothers who *do* manage schedules, return to work, raise other children, maintain a marriage, and travel. Today's women *are* able to fit breastfeeding into their lives. The ones who manage it best seem to be mothers who are willing to accept the special nature of their milk and the needs of their babies. Acknowledging these facts, they are able to make thoughtful decisions and workable arrangements for other aspects of their lives.

Women Tend to Feel Ambivalent about Breastfeeding

As we listened to women talking about nursing, it was clear that they experienced a variety of feelings. They spoke of what breastfeeding meant to them and to their babies in the physical sense. They also spoke of what it meant emotionally. Generally, new mothers expressed ambivalence about the experience, sometimes mentioning its value for the baby ("Is he getting enough milk?"), and often referring to the commitment it meant on their part. During some days—or hours—they could report feeling capable and content in their roles as nursing mothers. At other times, they might feel trapped and drained. As one mother explained about her first three months of nursing, "I had never felt so high and so low in my life."

A woman's attitude toward nursing seems to change as the weeks and months go by. For one thing, her focus changes. In the first weeks, she may be concerned with sore nipples and getting her baby to latch on properly and making enough milk. Once those issues are resolved, the mother is free to focus on others. In the second month, she may be more concerned with her milk leaking or with nursing in front of family and friends. By the third month, a nursing mother may be wondering about how to express or pump milk or how to have good sex again—or any sex again—even though she has full breasts and leaks milk and is too tired anyway. One mother, who nursed her daughter for a year, explained, "About once a month—like getting a period—I'd say, 'Why am I doing this?' I'd have all these complaints about my life, and I was sure they all revolved around breastfeeding. But then it would pass and I'd be so glad that I hadn't given it up."

If there are going to be negative reactions to nursing, it seems that they often come early on. That makes sense when you consider that the early weeks constitute a learning period for both mother and newborn. It must be said that some mothers find nursing enjoyable and problem-free from the beginning. "I was pleasantly surprised. It was much easier than I could have imagined." For others, however, the first weeks constitute what one mother called "that initial frightening period."

What seems frightening to some new mothers is the degree of dependence they recognize in their newborns. "I felt uncomfortable knowing he needed me that much." Another mother spoke of feeling overwhelmed by the seemingly incessant demands of a nursing newborn. "It depressed me. I was at her constant beck and call. I thought it would never end. I'd be chained to the house and would never be able to get dressed again." For some women, it can be difficult to believe that life as a nursing mother will ever become easier. "In the beginning I used to think, 'Why should I continue? I can't go anywhere. I can't do anything.' Now that I look back, the tough part was not that long. At the time, it seemed like forever." One woman explained that, as the weeks went by, she noticed a change in her own attitude. "At first I didn't realize that I could relax. I used to think, 'On, no. It's almost time to nurse.' Now I think, 'Oh, good. It's time to relax.'"

Ambivalent feelings make us feel uncomfortable. We want to make them go away. We often have the sense that if things were right or going well, there would be no ambivalence. There are several approaches to dealing with these mixed feelings about breastfeeding.

One approach might be to deny that there are any difficulties in the breastfeeding experience. Many of the earlier books on nursing did just this, suggesting a romantic picture of breastfeeding, entirely positive and uncomplicated.

A new approach suggests that, if any problems arise, there are quick and easy solutions. This thinking can lead mothers on a frantic search for the "right way" to breastfeed. The implication is that if we find the right way, both the problems and the ambivalence we feel will go away. An extension of this line of thinking could lead a new mother to conclude that if everything isn't going well, if she has any mixed feelings, she should give up breastfeeding.

We believe that although this ambivalence is uncomfortable and confusing, it is often part of being a parent. Throughout the process of loving and nurturing our children, we cannot deny that caring for them is work. Their needs will sometimes curtail our freedom and conflict with our own needs. Breastfeeding, as a parenting activity, is likely to produce these feelings of ambivalence. Such feelings exist even within the context of a satisfying nursing relationship. They are not necessarily a signal to give up breastfeeding.

In this book, when we describe a breastfeeding situation that has become difficult, we try to demonstrate how some information or support can help a new mother move beyond this point. It must be said, however, that sometimes information and support are not enough. For example, when job responsibilities are great, when other children are particularly demanding, or when separation from the baby is necessary, the unique requirements of breastfeeding may not fit into your life. Furthermore, if maintaining nursing in the face of continuing difficulty has become the single focus and the sole measurement of mothering, if it produces tension that distracts a woman from other important nurturing encounters, and if it interferes with her ability to enjoy her baby, a mother must reconsider her original decision to breastfeed. Whether to continue nursing your baby is a personal decision and should be based on what is best for you, your baby, and your family. Being a good mother does not depend upon your being a nursing mother.

If you choose to continue nursing, it will probably help if you can recognize the up-and-down nature of both motherhood and breastfeeding; if you can seek out information and hints from experienced mothers; and if you are able to get emotional support during this challenging time. We asked some women who had continued to nurse their babies beyond three months what they would like us to tell new mothers about breastfeeding. This is what they would like you to know:

I'd stress that you shouldn't be so hung up on schedules. Try to be flexible.

I must say it's a bit of an adjustment . . . give it time.

Keep telling yourself how healthy it is.

Understand that every baby is different. You have to learn from your baby what life is going to be like. Give to him freely . . . and your house will be happier.

Don't assume that everyone else who is nursing is crazy about it.

Just because you don't like some aspects of it doesn't mean you should give it up. Every job has parts you don't like.

When you're nursing your baby during those very early morning hours, you're not alone. Look out your window and know that other mothers are nursing and rocking wakeful babies.

Tell them that it gets better . . . it honestly does.

IT HONESTLY DOES.

2

The Early Days of Nursing

It takes six hands to breastfeed . . . the nurse's, my husband's, and my own.

—A NEW MOTHER

WHEN MANY of us think of a mother nursing her baby we picture a serene woman dressed in a loose, flowing robe sitting in a rocking chair with sunlight filtering in over her shoulder. She smiles as she looks down at her baby, who is nestled in her arms. We don't hear a sound as the mother slowly rocks back and forth, back and forth. The baby sucks noiselessly, then drops off to sleep.

This scene, without the flowing robe and filtered sunshine, probably occurs over and over for many nursing mothers. It may even occur in the first days of nursing. For many first-time mothers, however, the early period of nursing may not even faintly resemble this idyllic picture. As one mother of a three-day-old son said, "It takes six hands to breastfeed—the nurse's, my husband's, and my own."

The experiences of many women illustrate how uncertain the first weeks of mothering and nursing can be. Although the details of each story are unique, many women share circumstances that do not allow nursing to unfold according to a preconceived plan. Babies present challenges; hospital policies present obstacles; and the women's own feelings foster uncertainties. One or more of these areas caused problems for most of the women we met who were learning to nurse for the first time.

One woman who was a pediatrician and the mother of a six-week-old baby told us:

> Before I had Meredith, I used to look askance at mothers who said they stopped nursing because they didn't have enough milk. I knew every woman could produce enough milk for her baby. I thought in the back of my mind that mothers who didn't really want to nurse used that as an excuse. Well, once I had a baby I *felt* things differently.
>
> When Meredith was three weeks old, she fussed after every feeding and never seemed to settle down to sleep. She was miserable. I remember being convinced that she was not getting enough to eat. My factual knowledge didn't comfort me too much then. I depended on a friend who had had experience nursing. I forced myself to believe her words that Meredith was getting enough and that things would get smoother.

Another pediatrician who wholeheartedly supports breastfeeding said he always asks his prenatal patients if they plan to nurse. If they say yes, he says "Fantastic! But you know it's going to be hard." He has found that when mothers-to-be expect some difficulty, they manage to cope with the initial temporary problems without giving up nursing. He also explains that a nurse who works with him will visit during the first week at home. Thus the new mothers can have their confidence recharged by getting support and information at a time when they are likely to need it.

Some of the common *temporary* problems many women encounter as they begin to mother and nurse their babies, especially for the first time, include:

- Sleepy babies
- Fussy babies

- Babies who want to eat all the time
- Conflicting bits of advice
- Hospital policies that conflict with parents' wishes
- Worries about the techniques of nursing
- Worries about having enough milk
- Sore nipples
- Engorgement
- Feeling tired
- Feeling discouraged

Some of these concerns are directly related to learning to nurse. Many, however, are the result of adjusting to motherhood. Sore nipples, for example, are probably related to nursing, whereas feeling tired is probably related to mothering a newborn. It is important for you to realize that breastfeeding is not the root of all your difficulties. A husband or friend who understands breastfeeding can be a great ally. If your confidence wavers when well-meaning acquaintances suggest that all would be well if only you gave your baby some formula, you need someone to tell you that this is just not true.

Most mothers, even those who bottle-feed their babies, experience anxieties at first. Often the specific cause of the stress is not clear. Nevertheless, by six to eight weeks, most mothers and babies have settled into a mutually satisfying relationship, including relaxed nursing.

Dr. Derrick Jelliffe, a world-renowned authority on human milk and breastfeeding, has called successful nursing a "confidence trick." Despite the early questions and problems that arise, mothers have to maintain the belief that their babies will learn to nurse effectively. When confidence plummets and mothers get too anxious about their ability to nurse, lactation will be affected. A mother does best if she can develop a relaxed attitude, thinking of her baby as helping himself to milk. Both physiological *and* emotional factors influence how much milk is made and whether it "lets down" to be available for the baby.

If you are like most mothers, however, you may have trouble

maintaining that confidence on your own. You will need both the support and confidence of others and information about nursing. Whenever we asked a new mother how she managed the early weeks of adjustment, she invariably named someone she had depended upon for support. Frequently the person was her husband; often it was another woman who had had experience with nursing. The reassurance that things will get better may be all you will need. But you may need that reassurance many times a day.

Fundamentals of Breastfeeding

Your body has two tasks during nursing: making milk and giving it to the baby. In a way, the baby directs these processes because his sucking is crucial to each. When your baby sucks your nipple and the surrounding pigmented area called the areola, he stimulates the nerves that run from your breasts to parts of your brain. The sucking stimulation sends messages to your brain to release two hormones that are essential to lactation: prolactin and oxytocin. Prolactin controls milk production and oxytocin is associated with the let-down reflex.

Making Milk

When your baby is born, your body will experience a surge of prolactin as your placenta is expelled. The prolactin, carried by your bloodstream to your breasts, induces the glands in your breast to make milk from the nutrients within your body. After birth, any stimulation of your nipples increases the prolactin in the bloodstream. Sucking is the best way to increase prolactin, but even licking the nipple will do the same. Thus your baby's nursing is one of the best stimulants for milk production. When your baby nurses, your prolactin level rises and stays up for a short period of time. By three hours after the nursing has occurred, the prolactin level in your blood is back down to what it was before the baby was put to breast.

This suggests that frequent (more often than every three hours) nursing will keep the prolactin level up, thus increasing your milk supply. The more frequently the baby nurses, the more milk you will produce.

Besides controlling the amount of milk you produce, the frequency of nursing in the first days after birth also affects how quickly your milk will come in. When your baby is nursing soon after birth, then frequently thereafter, your milk is likely to come in within twenty-four to forty-eight hours. When your baby is nursing every three to four hours, on the other hand, your milk will probably come in after three to five days but may take up to a week.

How the mother experiences the milk's coming in varies from woman to woman. Within a few hours, your breasts may change from soft and empty to full and firm. Some mothers can tell exactly when this happens. For others it's a gradual process that occurs over several days or even weeks. Once your milk has come in, it increases markedly in the first few weeks in response to your baby's appetite. After the first few weeks, your supply is more stable.

Giving Milk

Producing milk is only half of your body's task. The milk is made in little glands called alveoli located throughout your breast. To be available for your baby, the milk must be ejected from the alveoli into the small collection pools or sacs just behind each nipple. The "milk ejection" or "let-down reflex" causes this to happen. When your baby sucks your nipple, a message is sent to your brain to release the hormone oxytocin. Oxytocin in turn travels to your breast and causes the cells around the alveoli to contract so that the milk is squeezed into the ducts that will carry it to the area near your nipple. This same hormone also causes your uterus to contract.

The let-down reflex has been called the main key to success or failure in lactation. Regardless of how much milk you produce, without the let-down reflex, you cannot give it to your baby. What is important about this reflex is that it is not automatic. It can be inhibited by anxiety, uncertainty, or other forms of emotional tension.

Furthermore, the let-down is a conditioned reflex. At first, it is triggered by your baby's sucking. In time (sometimes a very short time), it becomes linked to your baby and associations with him. Many mothers experience a let-down when the baby cries or when they are at work and someone asks about the baby. One mother said she always had one in the supermarket; the Ivory Snow was enough to trigger her let-down. If you are nursing a second or third baby, you may experience a let-down response sooner than a first-time nursing mother because your response has been conditioned in the past.

Before the response is conditioned, your baby usually must suck for a few minutes before the milk lets down. You may feel a warm, tingly, pins-and-needles sensation as the blood rushes into your breasts just before the let-down occurs. Or you may never feel any particular sensations at all. One of the best signs that your let-down response has occurred is when your baby, who has been sucking, suddenly starts to suck and *swallow*. Milk often will drip from your other breast, too, because the let-down occurs in both breasts at the same time.

One mother who had a strong let-down sensation said that when her two-week-old started sucking, then pulled away, he would get sprayed in the face. Months later she found milk on the rocking chair rungs. Her husband used to tease her that she could win "milk distance" contests. Although you may have a strong let-down, your milk does not have to spray across the room to be effective. All it has to do is get to the sacs behind your nipple. From there, it is your baby's responsibility to get it out.

The let-down response is exquisitely attuned to your feelings. That's why if you've had a premie and he's in the hospital, you may be so worried that your let-down response is inhibited. This anxiety makes pumping milk for premies especially difficult. Even if you've had a full-term baby, normal anxieties about your new role and how well you can breastfeed can interfere with your relaxing. Just being tired can inhibit your let-down response. This may be one reason why babies often nurse more frequently in the evening—they don't get enough milk after everyone's busy day. Unfortunately, a vicious cycle can emerge. You feel anxious, so your milk doesn't let down. Your baby gets frustrated and fusses, which is sure to increase your level of anxiety.

To prevent this vicious cycle from developing, try some of the following routines, which have helped other mothers to relax before nursing.

To encourage milk let-down, you should rub your nipples briskly but gently for a few minutes using your palm or fingers. Some women prefer a gentle, tickling stimulation of the nipples. When massaging is done correctly, the nipples should become erect and possibly tingle a bit, which can set off the let-down reflex.

If you are having difficulty getting a let-down response, Diana Stewart and Carol Gaiser, two nurses in a newborn nursery, recommend specific techniques before trying to express milk (pp. 49–51). Procedures such as the following promote let-down during both pumping and nursing:

• *Rest.* Lie down or sit with your feet up for ten to fifteen minutes to relax before you nurse. Some mothers choose a quiet place and, if at home, put on a favorite record, close their eyes, and try to think about how special their baby is.

• *Something to drink.* Find something good to drink to help you pause and interrupt the day's hectic pace. One mother reported treating herself to pretzels, cheese, and beer before her early evening nursing session.

• *Breathing.* Rhythmic, slow chest breathing is calming for some women.

• *Warmth.* Place hot, moist towels over your nipple, areola, breast, and surrounding tissue for about ten minutes before nursing. This will help you to relax and will also dilate your milk ducts to improve your milk flow. A hot shower or bath may do the same trick.

• *Massage.* A back rub between the shoulder blades, from which the nerves to the breast tissue radiate, can make nursing more effective by increasing circulation to the breast tissue. Also, gentle breast massage relieves tightness and increases circulation. Starting at the upper portion of the breasts, you should massage down toward the nipple. Small, circular motions help open the ducts. This massage is helpful both before nursing and, if you are pumping milk, before and during expression.

• *Syntocinon.* An oxytocin nasal spray prescribed by a physician can be helpful in stimulating milk let-down. If you use it before each nursing for a few days, the let-down will probably begin working on its own.

How Your Baby Sucks

The areola, or skin around your nipple, usually changes from a pinkish color before pregnancy to a reddish brown after. Some people have suggested that the areola is the same color as the nipple so that the baby will see and grasp both as he begins to suck. This is important because your baby's sucking consists of three motions. First, his jaws must squeeze the sinuses or milk-collection pools located beneath and just behind the areola. Then he sucks the milk into his mouth and swallows it.

Your baby milks the breast in this squeeze-suck-swallow, squeeze-suck-swallow rhythm. When he is actually sucking for milk, all the muscles of his face seem to be working together—even those near his temples.

One mother told us of the exceptionally good help she got from the two labor nurses who accompanied her new family to the recovery room to help begin nursing. She said the nurse helped the baby grasp the nipple and areola correctly by gently breaking the suction of the baby's grasp each time she got only the nipple in her mouth. They did this two or three times, saying, "No, Julie, you have to get more in your mouth." The nurses also wanted to be sure the nipple was on top of the baby's tongue because the baby must use the tongue both to hold the nipple against the top of her mouth and to stroke it during her squeeze-suck motions.

Putting the Baby to Breast

Many mothers-to-be are anxious about how the first nursing will go. As one mother in her ninth month of pregnancy told us, "I'm worried about the first time. Will my baby know how to nurse? It will be up to me. I've read, but I'm not sure if I'll know what to do. I know the first time is important. I know I have to be relaxed." As with any other skill to be learned, practice is necessary before a person feels confident. You may feel awkward putting your baby to breast the first time. How well the experience goes depends a lot on your baby. Some babies seem to know what to do right away, but others don't even know how to try.

Dr. George Barnes and his associates, who were at Yale a number of years ago and had had experience helping hundreds of mothers and babies get started nursing, classified babies by their feeding characteristics as barracudas, excited ineffectives, procrastinators, gourmets or mouthers, and resters. See if your baby seems to fit one of these patterns. You can expect your first nursing to be affected by his style.

BARRACUDAS. When put to the breast, barracudas vigorously and promptly grasp the nipple and suck energetically for from 10 to 20 minutes. There is no dallying. Occasionally this type of infant puts too much vigor into his nursing and hurts the nipple.

EXCITED INEFFECTIVES. These infants become so excited and active at the breast that they alternately grasp and lose the breast. They then start screaming. It is often necessary for the nurse or mother to pick up the infant and quiet him first, and then put him back to the breast. After a few days the mother and infant usually become adjusted.

PROCRASTINATORS. Procrastinators often seem to put off until the fourth or fifth postpartum day what they could just as well have done from the start. They wait till the milk comes in. They show no particular interest or ability in sucking in the first few days. It is important not to prod or force these infants when they seem disinclined. They do well once they start.

GOURMETS OR MOUTHERS. Gourmets insist on mouthing the nipple, tasting a little milk and then smacking their lips before starting to nurse. If the infant is hurried or prodded, he will become furious and start to scream. Otherwise, after a few minutes of mouthing he settles down and nurses very well.

RESTERS. Resters prefer to nurse a few minutes and then rest a few minutes. If left alone, they often nurse well, although the entire procedure will take much longer. They cannot be hurried (Barnes et al., pp. 194–96).

Regardless of which feeding style your baby shows, he has three reflexes that enable him to nurse: rooting, sucking, and swallowing. A newborn baby will *root* or turn his head toward anything that touches his cheek, mouth, or the skin around his mouth. So if your nipple touches your baby's left cheek, he will turn to the left and open his mouth to grasp the nipple. Once he has the nipple (or a finger) in his mouth, he will start to *suck*. If he gets anything, he will *swallow*. This means that at birth, your full-term baby is already programmed to get food when your breast is offered. Premature babies also have or will develop these skills. Babies who are born more than six weeks early sometimes must mature a little before they can smoothly produce and coordinate them (see Chapter 4).

Getting Comfortable

Many mothers find sitting up, either in a chair or in a bed with some back support, to be most comfortable at first. Since you will

want to take your time nursing, ask someone to put pillows anywhere you need extra support: behind your back, under the arm that
will support your baby, and maybe under your knees if you are in
bed. A pillow beneath your baby on your lap may help support his
weight comfortably and will bring him closer to your breast. Whatever position you choose, be sure the front of your baby's body is
facing yours. This way, he will not have to turn his head to the side
as he nurses and swallows. To see how uncomfortable that would
feel, turn your head to one side and then swallow.

When your baby starts mouthing or nuzzling for your breast, or
when you feel you are ready to try nursing him, use your arm that
is holding him (say, your left arm) to guide him toward your body.
Use your other hand (say, the right) to hold your breast for him.
Make a "V" sign with your right index finger and middle finger.
Turn your "V" sign sideways and place your fingers around your
areola. This helps to make the areola protrude and allows the baby
to latch on more easily.

If your baby is not already rooting for your nipple, touch his
cheek near his mouth with your nipple or finger. If he is not too
drowsy, he will turn, opening his mouth, and latch on. Ideally, he
will begin sucking and you will be on your way as a nursing couple.

The first times you nurse, it is important to be sure the baby's
mouth is closed on both your nipple *and* areola. Sheila Kitzinger in
The Experience of Breastfeeding has called this the "art of fixing" (p.
54). She quotes Chloe Fisher, a midwife tutor in Oxford, as saying
that a baby who has never been coaxed enough with the inviting
nipple may never open his mouth sufficiently to get a good grasp on
the breast. If your baby does not seem to grasp enough of the nipple
and areola for the nipple to be drawn into the back of his mouth,
you can gently coax him to open his mouth wide by touching each
side and then perhaps the top of his mouth with your nipple. As he
roots in these successive directions, he will open his mouth. Then
you can gently (but quickly!) insert your breast so his jaws close on
more than just the nipple as he starts to suck. This way, he is in the
proper position to carry out the squeeze-suck-swallow movements
necessary to empty your breast.

You can do a little experiment to feel the difference made when your baby has a good grasp. First, put your fingertip in your own mouth and suck. Then put your whole finger in your mouth and suck. You can feel how much more effective the sucking motions are when your whole finger is in your mouth. Less strain is exerted on the nipple when it is well back in the baby's mouth.

After a while on the first breast, you can break the suction by using your finger and pressing down on your breast near the corner of the baby's mouth. If the baby falls asleep on the first breast, you can wait a while before waking him to offer your second breast or you can wait for him to awaken on his own. Babies often like short, frequent feedings in the first days of life.

If you are more comfortable lying down, lie on one side (say, your left) with your left arm extended above your head. You may want a pillow behind your back or near your knees—anywhere you would like extra support. Place your baby in your bed on his side facing you. Pull him close with your right hand so your nipple barely touches his cheek. You can raise or lower your nipple by rolling your body slightly. If you tuck your baby's feet in toward your tummy, the angle of his body will keep his nose free to breathe.

When you are ready to change breasts, you can turn over without getting up by hugging your baby to you and turning over together before beginning again with your baby facing you on the other side. Or you can keep your baby where he is and just rotate your body so your right breast comes into contact with his mouth.

How Long to Nurse

There is a controversy about how long to nurse on each breast in the first days of nursing. Some feel the time should be restricted to prevent sore nipples. There is clear evidence, however, that some women never get sore nipples whereas others will get them whether or not the nursing time is restricted.

Information on how to reduce soreness begins on page 39.

Many authorities now agree that it is not useful to limit sucking time on either breast. It is important, however, if possible, to have the baby nurse from each breast. Some mothers encourage the baby to suck from both at each feeding. In other cases the baby alternates from one feeding to the next. Being sure the baby empties each breast (at the same or alternate feedings) will foster a good supply of milk.

Hospital Policies

When mothers give birth in hospitals, many of their early nursing experiences are shaped by hospital policies. Some hospitals have birthing rooms; others do not. Some allow parents to be with their babies in privacy soon after birth; others do not. Some hospitals have rooming-in or modified rooming-in arrangements so the baby can stay in the mother's room for extended periods of time; others keep the babies in central nurseries except for feedings every four hours. Some nursery staffs give babies formula or sugar water if they get fussy; others take the babies to their mothers. Some nursery staffs routinely weigh babies before and after breastfeeding to determine how much the baby has taken; others never do this. These policies can influence nursing by dictating when you get your baby, what happens when he is not with you, and how vital you're considered to be in his care. Remember that you often have a say in how these policies are carried out. Question the policies that don't support breastfeeding and ask for changes that will help you. Many pediatricians, for example, are willing to write orders directing the nursing staff not to give formula.

Some hospitals have postpartum nurses who give mothers tremendous support and accurate information for beginning breastfeeding; others have staff members who unwittingly undermine the mothers' efforts. Individual nurses and physicians vary tremendously in both their feelings about breastfeeding and their ability to help breastfeeding mothers. One mother recounted the following episode.

When my son Joseph was brought to me every four hours, he was always asleep. By the second day, the nurse who brought him announced to me, "This kid has got to eat. If he doesn't he'll get jaundice." She said if he wouldn't nurse, I'd have to give him formula. She hit him on his feet and she washed his face with cool water. Who could sleep through that? Joseph woke up and started to suck. The nurse was very strict about allowing only three or four minutes on each side. She told me if I went longer I'd get sore nipples and then I'd be in terrible shape. I was a little confused, because Joseph would fall asleep nursing on one side, but he'd keep sucking while he was sleeping. I knew the sucking was good for bringing in milk. If I took him off one breast to switch him to the other, he would stop sucking and would not latch on to the other breast.

When nurses or doctors speak with conviction, it's hard to evaluate what they are saying. This mother knew that the nurse's directions were not helping her get nursing established. Joseph clearly was not on a four-hour schedule. He was probably waking up after short intervals of sleep, ready to nurse. If his mother had been with him, she could follow his rhythms and feed him when he showed signs of hunger. The mother also noticed that limiting Joseph's time on each breast seemed to inhibit his sucking. She already knew her baby better than the nurse did. She was becoming the expert about her baby despite others' professional training.

If you are hearing admonitions and restrictions that don't seem to work with your baby, share your observations with the staff. If they don't seem to hear, just remember they do not necessarily know best. Test your ideas, share them with your husband or friend, and if you can't use them in the hospital, save them for when you go home.

Unfortunately, you may face a dilemma while you're in the hospital. On one hand, you may disagree with the policies that dictate when and how long you will have your baby. On the other hand, if you get too worked up over issues beyond your control, your own anxiety may interfere with nursing. Sometimes your husband can play an important role as intermediary between you and the hospital personnel, especially when practices are dictated less by policy than by convenience. We heard story after story of fathers actively intervening in ways that helped their partners with nursing.

For example, one mother, Barbara Ferguson, told us that she was becoming frustrated and exasperated in the hospital because each time she received her baby for a feeding a nurse was also present "to help." The mother could not relax with her baby and take her time in privacy. The nurse was aggressive in her attempts to get the baby successfully latched on. By the end of the second day, breastfeeding still was not working.

Barbara called her husband and explained that she wanted *him* to bring her the baby for the next feeding. She wanted no nurses and no instruction. Bob Ferguson arrived at the hospital and arranged to bring his daughter to Barbara. He handed the baby to his wife, pulled the curtain around the three of them, and Barbara began nursing. She claims she felt happy, relaxed, and comfortable. Nursing was working.

If your hospital's practices offer you choices about issues such as nursing in the first hour or rooming-in, it is important to be informed about the options so that you can choose arrangements that will foster breastfeeding. If options are not available, you should remember that successful lactation can occur even after less-than-ideal beginnings. The ingredients to strive for are relaxation and plenty of breast stimulation. Sucking is the best source of stimulation, but even your baby's licking or touching the nipple will help bring in your milk.

Nursing Soon after Giving Birth

After having labored and given birth, many mothers are in limbo—savoring the deliciousness of their work being over. Feeling exhausted is common, in addition to feeling relieved that it is all finally over. Giving birth is like climbing a mountain. Once you have climbed up, you have to climb down. Not only are you in for the duration, you also will have to play an active role. So, once the job is over, most mothers are spent. Many told us how listless they felt. Many said they did not even care about seeing or holding their babies right away. They were concerned about themselves.

Yet when the baby is put in their arms, mothers are often captivated. As one mother said, "I was so tired, I never would have asked for Lisa. But once I had her, I couldn't let her go." "When she looked at me, I knew she was mine," reminisced another. Feelings of elation often fill new parents as they take in their little one. His eyes, his skin, his little fingers and toes, his cry, his gaze—everything about him becomes a source of wonder.

Drs. Marshall Klaus and John Kennell, pediatricians and authors, have identified the minutes and hours after birth as a time when you are especially sensitive to the exquisite features of your new baby. Primed by nine months of pregnancy and your recent experiences of labor and birth, you are uniquely ready to become attached to your young.

Complementing your interest in the behavior of your newborn soon after birth, he is more likely to be alert and attentive in those first forty-five minutes than he will be at any time in the next twelve hours. He is also likely to suck well if you were not sedated during labor or birth. Thus the first hour or so is a wonderful time to meet. Your interest in your baby's eyes is likely to be met by his wide-eyed gaze. Your interest in nursing may well be rewarded by your baby's being awake and capable of rooting and sucking eagerly.

If you first have contact when you're both ready to respond, your interactions are likely to be mutually rewarding. This is especially important if you are inexperienced. You can remember how alert your baby can be when he goes into a sleepy state and can no longer be awakened to nurse. Babies are often very sleepy the second and third days of life.

How your baby responds to your first nursing attempts is likely to color your view of how breastfeeding will go. This can be seen in the contrasting statements of two mothers, one of whom nursed within the first hour and the other at sixteen hours. The first mother told us, "I put my baby to breast in the recovery room. She seemed to know what to do. She did better than I did!" The mother who first nursed at sixteen hours postpartum lamented, "My baby's less than twenty-four hours old, so we'll give nursing a whirl. But I don't know. My baby's sleepy. My breast seems to put her to sleep." This mother didn't realize that everything puts the one- or two-day-old baby to sleep. Or more precisely, nothing wakes him up. Not all mothers are high in the first hour, and not all babies are alert. Yet many are. So being together during that time is like stacking the deck in favor of a comfortable first meeting.

That is not to say, however, that it is necessary to be together and nurse in the first hour. Many mothers and babies have wonderful nursing relationships that began hours, days, or even weeks (if the baby was born prematurely) after birth. Dr. Betsy Lozoff, a pediatrician who has done cross-cultural research, has suggested that in our culture, in which babies are relatively deprived of bodily contact during the first year of life, contact in the first hour has taken on added significance. In many nonindustrialized societies, babies are held virtually all the time; they are carried during the day and sleep with parents or siblings at night. American babies, in contrast, are usually held only briefly and expected to sleep alone from birth. Perhaps parents who get to hold their babies soon after birth find the experience so wonderful that they want to hold their babies a lot. Maybe the experience seems so important because it changes how parents feel about having their babies nearby. Customs of child care are changing here, however, so that many parents are providing increased bodily contact with their babies regardless of their early postpartum experience.

Early Feeding Schedules

While you are in the hospital, how often you get the chance to feed your baby will depend largely on the hospital's rooming arrangements for you and your baby. Some hospitals still keep babies in central nurseries and bring them to mothers for feeding every four hours. In others, babies stay with their mothers for larger blocks of time—all afternoon, all day, or sometimes all day and night. It is best if you have your baby with you for hours at a time so you can nurse him whenever either of you is interested. In one hospital that encourages mothers to feed their babies as often as they wish, feedings occur anywhere from seven to twenty-five times a day. Feeding as often as every hour or hour and a half is not uncommon. Nor is it unusual for the baby to nurse and fall asleep on one breast, then wake up forty-five minutes later to nurse from the other. When mothers and babies are given the freedom to nurse, they usually develop individual patterns, including frequent feedings.

If your baby is very sleepy and *you* set the feeding times, pick him up and offer your breast at least every two or three hours. We usually think of a baby showing his hunger by crying, but this is probably his last resort. If you watch your sleepy baby, you may notice that at times he becomes restless, stretches, mouths, or even brings his hand or fingers up to his mouth to suck. These may be his early signals of hunger.

There are many advantages to nursing frequently in the first days. The abundant sucking stimulation will help to bring in your milk sooner and to increase your milk supply. Before your milk comes in, your breasts are filled with colostrum, which is a wonderful source of protein and antibodies for your baby. Your baby will benefit by sucking every drop of colostrum he can get. You will benefit from his removing all the colostrum because then the ducts or small channels in your breasts will be emptied. This is likely to decrease the possibility of your breasts becoming overfull or engorged when your milk does come in.

Frequent nursing will also help prevent sore nipples. Breastmilk is so digestible that the baby's stomach is usually empty after one and one-half hours. If he has to wait three or four hours to feed, he is more likely to be very hungry and therefore chomp down and suck aggressively. If you do get sore nipples, frequent short nursings can help you cope until the soreness goes away.

Feeding frequently or on demand is also the best way to assure that your baby will be ready to suck when you try to nurse. Babies will suck more vigorously when they're allowed to awaken by themselves. If your baby is brought to you every four hours according to the nursery's feeding schedule, he may not be awake or hungry when you try to nurse. So no matter what you do, he may feed poorly or not at all. If this is how feeding is arranged in the hospital where you have your baby and your requests for a change have been denied, try to relax and keep telling yourself that once you get home, you can start feeding more frequently.

Supplementary Bottles

Linked to the question of feeding schedules is the issue of giving supplementary bottles of water, sugar water, or formula.

If you are feeding your baby on demand, there is no reason for him to have supplementary bottles. Colostrum is all your baby needs until your milk comes in. Throughout most of human existence, there were no plastic or glass bottles, no rubber or vinyl nipples, no formula. Newborns not only survived; they thrived solely on mother's milk. If you're feeding frequently, your milk will come in sooner.

If your baby is brought to you only every four hours because of fixed hospital policies, he may become so hungry between feedings that he gets frantic. Try to persuade the nurses to let you fetch him from the nursery before that happens. If you cannot, your baby will probably be more comfortable if he has a little something to hold him over. Water or sugar water is better than formula in those cases, because water is less likely to fill him up and does not predispose him to allergies. If your hospital has a rigid feeding schedule, however, the question of whether your baby gets supplements may be beyond your control. Asking your doctor to write an order specifying no formula may help. If not, remember you can stop the supplements as soon as you get home.

Once home, it is best to avoid supplementary bottles whenever possible because sucking an artificial nipple is easier for your baby than sucking from your breast. Because the milk pours out of the hole in the artificial nipple, the baby's main task is to stop the flow by pushing the nipple against the roof of his mouth with his tongue. *This is very different from the squeeze-suck-swallow actions involved in nursing.* Babies who are given too many bottles before nursing is established show much less vigorous sucking at the breast. When this happens, the mother's breast gets less of that essential sucking stimulation. So, if possible, avoid bottles for at least six to eight weeks. The exception is if you plan to return to work early. Mothers report having more success getting their babies to take bottles if they are introduced early. If you need to use a supplementary bottle, perhaps your husband can give your baby one or two bottles a week from the first or second week.

Sore Nipples

Sore nipples are very common early in nursing. Usually the soreness goes away sometime between two days and two weeks. While it lasts, though, it can seem unbearable. One mother of four said she used to send her older children out of the room when she began nursing her youngest because tears streamed down her face whenever he latched on. Mothers nursing a second or third child often report the pain to be much worse than it was with their first babies. It also seems to be worse for blondes and redheads with fair skin.

The "toe-curling" pain sometimes described by mothers usually occurs as the baby first latches on for each feeding. It usually lasts only until the milk lets down. In the first days of nursing, this may take a couple of minutes, but as the let-down becomes conditioned, it may occur just seconds after the baby starts sucking. Some women do their Lamaze breathing to get through these minutes or seconds. Nipple soreness diminishes by itself with time. There are, however, some measures you can take to help along its demise.

• Be sure the baby is fixed well on your breast for each feeding. He should take all of the nipple and much of the areola into his mouth during his squeeze-suck-swallow action.

• Nurse frequently so your baby is not frantic for food. A famished baby will suck much more aggressively than one who is just beginning to feel hunger.

• Nurse for at least several minutes on each breast. Contrary to some common advice, limited feedings may aggravate the problem if the baby is taken from your breast before your milk has let down. Since the pain is likely to diminish once the let-down response has occurred, you are both likely to enjoy your nursing experience if you continue long enough.

• If your let-down response seems to take a long time to occur, stimulate your breast by massaging it and manually expressing some milk *before* your baby begins to suck. Other clues for stimulating the let-down response were given earlier in this chapter.

• Offer your baby the breast with the less sore nipple first because the let-down will occur in both breasts at once. Thus the vigorous initial sucking will be on the less painful side.

• Never pull your baby off your breast. If he does not let go of the breast when he finishes nursing, break the suction by pressing down on your breast near the corner of his mouth before removing him.

• Vary your positions for nursing. The pressure points on your breast occur where his tongue strokes it and where the two corners of his mouth clamp down. If you vary how you hold him during nursing (for example, sitting with his body across your lap; using the football hold with his body beneath your underarm), the points on your breast where his tongue and mouth corners exert pressure will also change.

• Always allow your nipples to air dry after nursing because moisture increases the soreness and growth of bacteria. Avoid bras or bra pads with plastic liners, which will prevent the nipples from drying. Short exposure to direct sunshine will also help the healing process. Warm air from a hair dryer may also help.

• Never use soap or alcohol on your nipples because they remove the natural secretions that keep the nipples soft and pliable and protect them from the irritations of the baby's sucking. You can also rub vitamin E oil or pure hydrous lanolin into your nipple and areola after feeding to augment the natural secretions. If you are allergic to wheat, you should not use vitamin E oil that is derived from wheat germ, and if you are allergic to wool, avoid lanolin, which comes from sheep.

• Some women have found that their nipples heal more quickly if they apply a little of their own breastmilk after nursing and allow the nipples to air dry. Breastmilk contains antibodies, and in some cultures, it is dropped in babies' eyes to cure eye infections.

• Finally, be forewarned that unless your doctor is experienced in supporting mothers during breastfeeding, he or she may suggest that you give your baby a bottle if you complain of sore nipples. Doing this is likely to disrupt your attempts to establish nursing.

Engorgement

When your milk first comes in, sometime within the first two to five days after giving birth, your breasts are likely to feel full. This is because the milk is filling the alveoli and there is an increased flow of blood and lymph to your breasts. If your breasts become overfilled (hard, painful, and warm to the touch), you are engorged. Engorged breasts can be terribly painful. They can be as hard as grapefruits and tender to the slightest touch. All new mothers experience some fullness, but not all become engorged. The probability of engorgement decreases with each successive child.

The best treatment for engorgement is prevention. The best prevention is to nurse your baby frequently both day and night from the day of birth. This will keep your breasts empty and decrease the possibility of the milk's accumulating without being removed. The chance of your becoming engorged will be greatest if you feed your baby on a four-hour schedule. If your hospital allows no flexibility on this issue, try to nurse your baby at the beginning and end of your times together. Also, ask to be awakened to nurse him at night.

If you do become engorged, remember it is only a temporary condition and not a permanent part of breastfeeding. Even without any intervention, your breasts will get softer and smaller in twenty-four to forty-eight hours. In the meantime, there are some comfort measures you can try. The purpose of these is to soften your breasts, both to relieve your discomfort and to make your nipple and areolar area soft enough for your baby to grasp. It is important that your baby empty your breasts so milk production will continue. If the milk backs up in your breasts, a message is sent to your brain to stop producing it. Remember that your milk supply is based on demand.

• Apply heat to your breasts for ten to twenty minutes before nursing. You can use warm wash cloths, submerge your breasts in a basin of warm water, or take a warm shower. If you take a shower, stand with your back to the water and let it run over your shoulders down your breasts. While doing this, you can use one hand to support one breast at a time and the other to stroke downward away from your shoulder and underarm toward your nipple. The warmth will relax your tissues, and the massaging is likely to begin the milk flow, thereby removing some of the fullness.

• If your baby has trouble grasping your nipple and areola, gently massage those areas and hand express some milk before he is ready to nurse. Five minutes of massage on each breast is usually adequate even if your milk is not dripping. Then use your fingers in a "V" sign to grasp your breast around your areola so your baby can fix properly. If your baby grasps and sucks only your nipple, you will find it very painful. Besides, your baby must fix well on your nipple and areola so as to milk your breast sufficiently to empty the ducts. Without adequate emptying, your breasts will stay full and your baby will be frustrated by not getting enough milk.

• Change your baby's nursing position to empty all parts of your breasts.

• After nursing, some mothers find cold packs applied to the breasts reduce the swelling and pain. Some find alternating hot and cold packs to be soothing.

• Wear a well-fitting bra with wide straps (so your shoulders are not cut by the weight of your breasts) twenty-four hours a day. The support provided will alleviate some of the tenderness you feel.

• Ask your physician for an aspirin or aspirin-codeine preparation if you need more pain relief. These will not harm your nursing baby (Lawrence, p. 221).

• Nurse very frequently from both breasts at each feeding as long as your engorgement lasts.

Stay with it. Even without any of these comfort measures, the swelling will go down within a couple of days. When it does, your breasts may seem empty. They are not! You have not lost your milk. Your body has merely accomplished the feat of adjusting to milk production. Congratulations!

Reality Changes

The lovely image of breastfeeding conjured up in the beginning of this chapter seems a far cry from the reality of the first weeks of nursing. Engorged breasts or sore nipples are not the stuff of which dreams are made. Breastfeeding, like pregnancy and parenting, may never be idyllic. But the reality of breastfeeding does change. It gets easier and less uncomfortable as your body, your emotions, and your baby adjust. Mothers and babies, in fact, really come to enjoy it.

3

Nursing After a Cesarean Birth

*I felt so needed when Robby
was calmed by nursing, and
feeling needed was really
important to me then.*

—A NEW MOTHER after a
Cesarean birth experience

BEGINNING to breastfeed your baby after a Cesarean childbirth is similar to beginning to nurse after a vaginal birth. The principles of breastfeeding remain the same. In the long run, your Cesarean delivery will not affect your milk supply, let-down reflex, the length of time your milk takes to come in, or your baby's desire to nurse. Your body starts producing milk when you deliver your baby and the placenta. The birth of the placenta, in particular, triggers a surge of hormones that begins the process. Whether the birth is through the vagina or an abdominal incision does not make any difference. Your body is primed to nurse.

The primary difference is that you are likely to feel incisional pain and discomfort from surgery for the first days, or even weeks, after giving birth. As one mother said, "I hurt when I got out of bed, I hurt when I coughed, I hurt when I laughed. It took a few weeks until getting up didn't make my stitches hurt." You may have trouble getting comfortable holding your baby, and you may feel apprehensive about the contact that nursing entails. Yet several mothers we interviewed commented spontaneously that they felt better—actually experienced less pain—when their babies were with them.

Joni Smith, who gave birth to Megan, a nine-pound girl, by Cesarean birth after a twenty-four-hour labor, told us, "In the hospital I wanted Megan with me all the time. I felt funny asking the nurses to bring her. She wasn't crying or unhappy in the nursery, but I still wanted her. I liked holding her and nursing her. They thought I needed to rest. But when she wasn't with me, I felt so depressed. I felt lousy—like it hadn't been worth it. But when she was there, I felt okay."

Another mother said she was entertained by watching, touching, and nursing her baby. "As long as Tony was there, I didn't feel the pain as much. You don't pay attention to it the same way as when you're alone." This mother went on to explain, "I could barely walk the first two days. I got bad gas pains the second day, but none of that stopped my nursing."

These mothers suggest that recovering from their Cesareans caused discomfort for themselves but did not cause any particular problems with nursing—so long as the mothers had help getting their babies and getting as comfortable as possible with them, especially in the first days after birth. This chapter discusses how mothers can increase their comfort during breastfeeding by making optimal hospital arrangements, finding suitable nursing positions, and considering the use of pain medication and other relaxation measures.

Hospital Policies

Hospitals often have special rules for the care of mother, father, and baby following a Cesarean birth. Some of these rules can affect the ease or difficulty of your initial breastfeeding experiences.

• If your husband is permitted to be present for the Cesarean birth of your baby, his presence can help you feel positive about the birth. His involvement with both of you can be an important source of support for later breastfeeding.

• If your baby is permitted to go to the recovery room with you, you might try nursing him there before the effects of your anesthesia wear off.

• If your newborn is to be taken to the nursery for observation, maybe your husband can go with him and spend time holding him. Perhaps he can then arrange to bring the baby to you in the recovery room.

• If your baby can room in with you or stay with you for extended periods of the day, it will be easier for you to tell when he's ready to nurse. It will also give you more frequent and more relaxed opportunities to learn about nursing your infant.

• If your baby is staying in the nursery, maybe you can make arrangements for your husband to bring him to you whenever he visits. Many hospitals permit the father extended or unlimited visiting hours.

• If your husband is not available, perhaps you could arrange for a friend or relative to have extended visiting hours. A close friend or relative can be a wonderful source of physical and moral support as you try to nurse and care for your baby while still recovering from surgery. An extra pair of hands can be invaluable.

Hospital policies are not always ironclad. Practices may be matters of convenience rather than formalized rules. If you and your husband speak up, you may discover areas of flexibility conducive to breastfeeding. As a rule of thumb, the more time your husband, baby, and even other children can be with you during your first days after birth, the easier your adjustment will be.

Finding a Comfortable Position for Nursing

Once arrangements have been made to have your baby with you, your next job will be finding out how you are most comfortable nursing. The following positions are the ones described most favorably by mothers who have given birth by Cesarean.

If you have the opportunity to nurse your baby in the recovery room, try placing your baby prone across your chest so you stay flat on your back. Ask your husband or a nurse to stay next to you to help you support your baby in that position and help him accept your breast. You may be more comfortable raising one knee slightly. If your baby is awake, he may latch on and nurse. Even if he doesn't suck, his touching your nipple with his lips—or tasting or licking it—will trigger a rise of prolactin in your body which is essential for producing milk.

Most mothers report that during the first day or two, they nurse their babies lying in bed with the top of the bed elevated slightly. You may be most comfortable lying sideways with your back against the guardrail and cushioned with pillows. To nurse lying down, follow the instructions on page 31. Remember to have someone tuck pillows around you for support. Some mothers like to have a pillow placed under the baby to lift him to the height of the nipple. Although this position is frequently used, many mothers feel increased incisional pain from the pressure of the abdomen pulling to one side. If this is true for you, ask a nurse to tuck a pillow or bath blanket under your abdomen to help support it.

Many mothers find sitting straight up in bed or in a chair, as described on page 29, to be best for them. Place a stool or overturned bath basin covered with a pillow under your feet to provide support for your legs and prevent extra stretching of your abdominal muscles. Have a pillow placed under the arm that supports your baby to help you relax your arm and shoulder muscles. Another pillow over your abdomen will raise the baby to the height of your breast and protect your incision.

A few mothers prefer to sit tailor fashion on a bed with the baby lying on a pillow across their knees. If you lean forward slightly, there will be little weight on your incision. Remember to keep your shoulders relaxed, so that you will not tire yourself.

A third variation on the sitting position is the football hold. To feed your baby from your left breast, for example, hold the baby's head near your breast cupped in your left palm with the baby's body extending around your left side beneath your armpit. You can support your left arm and the baby on a pillow or two. In this position, the baby's body does not lie across your abdomen.

Be sure to ask for help in positioning and repositioning your baby. Treat yourself to the extra hands so you can enjoy your first opportunities to see, smell, touch, explore, and nurse your newborn. You will feel better and need less help with each passing day. Give in to your early awkwardness and get the help you need to minimize your physical discomfort.

Pain Medication

Although the rule of thumb for breastfeeding mothers is to avoid unnecessary medication, most mothers who have had a Cesarean birth find that small doses of pain medicine help them manage during their first postoperative days. As one Cesarean breastfeeding mother who is also a pediatrician said, "The analgesia takes the edge off the pain so you can move around. Otherwise, the thought of finding a comfortable position for breastfeeding would be unbearable for the first few days. And you surely don't want mothers to wait three or four days before beginning to nurse."

When a breastfeeding mother takes drugs, she may be concerned whether the drug passes into the breastmilk and, if so, whether it affects the baby. Unfortunately, the research on these issues is often outdated and incomplete. Yet certain pain medications have been used widely by breastfeeding mothers without adverse effects on the baby. Just be sure that your doctor knows you are breastfeeding or that you plan to breastfeed, so he or she can prescribe one of the analgesics thought to be safe for your baby.

To help you avoid the potential risks associated with pain medication, nurse the baby immediately before or after taking oral pain medicine and immediately before an injection. Theoretically, the level of medicine in your milk should be lowest with this timing. Some drugs pass into your breastmilk only in small quantities, yet the cumulative effect over a twenty-four-hour period could equal a full dose for your baby. Therefore, you should be aware of the size of the dosage you are taking and the length of time you are taking it. Again, you might ask your doctor to prescribe the lowest adequate dose at first. Then he or she can prescribe more if that dose is insufficient. As you're feeling better, ask to have the dosage reduced. Don't take the drugs longer than necessary. As alternative ways of coping with pain, try moving around frequently, use relaxation techniques, and spend time with your baby.

Babies who are unusually sleepy or irritable or who exhibit vomiting or diarrhea may be showing signs of being hypersensitive to your medication. If your baby has problems after birth, ask your pediatrician whether your pain medication could be contributing to your baby's condition.

Other Comfort Measures and Nursing Tips

• Drink plenty of liquids to counteract postoperative dehydration and increase your milk supply. You can drink liquids while on an IV.

• If your baby is to be separated from you for more than twenty-four hours, try pumping your breasts, as described in Chapter 4, to stimulate your milk production. You can successfully breastfeed even if you must wait a few days to initiate it. Pumping is important in the interim.

• Get out of bed as soon as you can and force yourself to walk. Although moving may be uncomfortable, the results of staying in one position too long will be worse.

• To help overcome gas pains, walk as much as you can and try doing abdominal tightening exercises.

• Ask a nurse to teach you how to lift your baby using your shoulder and back muscles while keeping your abdominals relaxed.

• Keep the side rails on your bed up to help you move around and switch sides during nursing.

• Ask for an electric bed you can adjust by yourself rather than one that is cranked manually.

• If you plan to have a roommate, ask if you might be placed in a room with another woman who has had a Cesarean. Much of the best advice and reassurance can come from another mother who shares your situation.

Once you go home, it is important to ask for and accept help with household tasks, so you can devote yourself to your baby and establish your nursing relationship. As one mother said, "When people leave you after a week—your mother goes home, your husband returns to work—you must say, 'I still need help.' "

Fatigue is the worst culprit in the weeks and even months after birth. Take care of yourself. Give yourself time to recover.

Some couples who have had an unexpected Cesarean birth feel very let-down afterward. Despite having a beautiful, healthy baby, mothers and fathers often feel disappointed for having missed the active vaginal birth for which they had prepared. If you or your husband feels inexplicably depressed or resentful, you might want to contact a Cesarean support group in your area. Talking with other parents who have had similar experiences may help you realize and come to terms with the pent-up feelings you have been experiencing.

Many women we met reported that their satisfaction with breastfeeding helped compensate for their disappointment about having had their babies by Cesarean. One mother said she had counted on having a prepared birth with little or no medication. "It had become part of my self-image," she explained. "When I had to have a Cesarean, I felt terrible. Why hadn't my body worked right?" She went on to describe how nursing had gone so well that it helped to restore her self-confidence. She was proud of how well her body could sustain her baby.

In addition to restoring confidence, breastfeeding can affect women's feelings about Cesareans in another important way. Breastfeeding completes the pregnancy-birth cycle; it rounds off the childbearing year. And once that year is over, the mother who is looking back often comes to realize that breastfeeding has had much more to do with nurturing and parenting than did the style of giving birth.

4

When Your Baby Comes Early

I didn't mind pumping after the first few aggravating episodes. In fact, I saw it was a means of bringing Rachael something.

—A NEW MOTHER

IF YOUR BABY is born prematurely, or less than thirty-seven weeks after conception, he will probably be taken to a special care nursery so the doctors and nurses can observe how he is doing. If he was just a little early and has no other problems, he may be returned to the full-term nursery and discharged from the hospital with you. In these instances, your experiences learning to breastfeed will be similar to those of the full-term mother described in Chapter 2, except that your premie is likely to be a sleepy baby at first.

If, on the other hand, your baby is born small (less than about four pounds) and/or has any problems, he will probably be hospitalized in an intensive care nursery until you can take him home. In most cases, you will still be able to breastfeed. You may have to wait awhile, however, until your baby is ready to begin nursing. In the meantime, it is important for you to build and maintain your milk supply by expressing the milk from your breasts.

Breastfeeding the Premature Baby

Your baby's gestational age (number of weeks since conception), size, and medical condition will influence both his behavior and his ability to begin nursing. Young premies (less than about thirty-two to thirty-five weeks) are still quite immature. Your premie's first task is to establish a physiological equilibrium: to develop stable breathing and sleeping patterns, to maintain body temperature, to absorb enough calories through his intestines, and to gain control of his often jerky body movements. In the days or weeks before these systems mature, your baby may not be able to handle too much extra stimulation. He may love being held close and cuddled but get fussy or turn red after prolonged face-to-face play. As he matures, however, he will be able to stay alert and enjoy increasingly long social encounters with you.

At about thirty-four weeks gestational age, your baby will be able to coordinate his sucking and swallowing responses. Before this age, he will not be able to nurse or even suck milk from a bottle. He will be fed milk through a small tube that is inserted through his nose into his stomach. As your baby matures and learns to take a nipple, he will probably be fed first from a bottle with a soft premie nipple that allows milk to flow easily. Often the transition from tube feeding (called *gavage*) to nippling is gradual, giving the baby time and experience to master the new technique. Since babies use more energy sucking from a premie nipple than while being gavage fed (and still more while nursing!), their behavior and weight gain are monitored as each change in feeding method is attempted.

Different nurseries have different policies about when they encourage mothers to put their babies to breast. In some nurseries, mothers try soon after the baby can suck well from a bottle. In others, the baby must reach a certain weight, often four pounds. Some nurseries do not have explicit rules. Instead, the doctors and nurses make individual decisions for each infant. The medical staff will consider such factors as how healthy the baby is, how stable his condition has been, whether he is still attached to monitors or machines, how well he's been gaining weight, how well he can maintain his body temperature during feeding, and whether he can continue to gain weight when using energy both to keep warm and to suck from the breast. Depending on these factors, you may be able to begin nursing within days after birth or you may have to wait weeks or even months. Even when your baby begins nursing at the breast, he may not be able to give up the bottle completely right away. Again, his weight gain and health will be watched as he moves from one to two to three nursings a day.

You do not have to wait to provide breastmilk for your baby. Breastmilk is considered to be the food of choice for most premature infants, even when they are being tube-fed. Therefore, mothers are encouraged to begin expressing their own milk and to bring it to the nursery for their babies as soon as they can. Since a breast pump cannot stimulate your breasts as well as your baby's sucking would, you may not produce enough milk to fulfill all your baby's nutritional requirements. His feedings may be supplemented with breastmilk from a donor or with formula. Nonetheless, whatever milk you produce is extremely valuable for your child.

If your premature infant is too small to nurse at birth and you plan to breastfeed, you must maintain your milk supply until you can actually put him to breast. You do this by emptying your breasts frequently with the help of a breast pump. Even mothers who do not plan to nurse are encouraged by doctors to express their milk for their babies because of the benefits of breastmilk. Certain properties of breastmilk are especially important for premies. Furthermore, your baby will benefit most from *your* own milk.

Why Your Milk Is Best for Your Baby

Because human milk is so good for premies, many hospitals maintain milk banks where breastmilk from many lactating mothers is stored. Although this milk is good for the baby, recent studies show that the baby's own mother's milk is best for him. The milk you produce on the third day of lactation is different from that you will produce one month later. The composition of your milk changes in keeping with the changing needs of your developing baby. For example, the amount of protein in the milk decreases from day three to day twenty-eight, and the amount of fat increases. Milk pooled from mothers at all stages of lactation will not show these changes in composition.

Furthermore, the milk you produce is different from the milk produced by mothers of full-term babies in that it has higher concentrations of protein, sodium, and chloride and lower concentrations of lactose. It is better suited to the nutritional needs of the premature infant. Since your milk is so well suited to your baby, any amount you can supply will be extremely beneficial for him.

Many mothers reported a deep sense of satisfaction in being able to provide this milk for their babies. One mother commented, "It's so good to see David grow and look so healthy. And I know it's because of me." Yet finding time to pump is no easy task. There you are separated from your baby, who lives in a busy nursery, your other children (if you have any) want you at home, your husband is probably feeling pressure from work, everyone is tired and maybe worried, too. And your job is to relax and pump milk for your baby. It is amazing any women manage to pump at all!

The first thing to remember is that you do not have to provide milk for your baby's survival. As good as your milk is, there are substitutes. Second, whatever small amount you can provide will be valuable. You do not have to pump enough to sustain your baby. Third, you do not have to pump for a specified period of time. If you can provide even your colostrum, you will be giving your baby a feast of antibodies. But, as discussed in Chapter 1, this is no contest. You can stop any time. Some mothers just pump while they are on the postpartum unit and someone else is taking care of their everyday responsibilities. You are an adult, a mother, a wife, and perhaps a career woman. You have many responsibilities. You must decide how to balance them. Breastfeeding your baby is not essential. It is part of the whole complex of relationships and interrelationships that make up your marriage, your family, your life.

Some women manage to pump for the first few weeks, when breastmilk is most important for their premies by saying, "This is what is important now. What other responsibilities can I ignore or pass on to somebody else for a while?" This is the time you need to call on your family and friends. Who can you ask to drive you to the hospital, cook some meals, run some errands? What jobs can you put off for two weeks? People often want to do something for the family of a hospitalized baby, but they feel too awkward to ask. Friends may feel they are bothering you if they call when you're coping with so much. They will appreciate your suggestions as to how to show their concern and support.

The rest of this chapter will provide practical information about the kinds of pumps available, the techniques of pumping, fostering a let-down response, scheduling, and so on. It will also describe the ways other mothers of premies have managed to learn to breastfeed among the concerns and demands of having a baby born early.

Expressing Breastmilk

Choice of Pumps

Before you can nurse your baby, you can express or pump your milk for him. This provides him with the benefits of your milk and also helps to build and maintain your milk supply. Since your breasts produce milk according to the law of supply and demand, they must be emptied before they will fill up with milk again. Until your baby can empty your breasts by nursing, you can do it by pumping. When the milk stays in your breast, it causes a back pressure within the milk ducts, which signals your body to stop producing milk. When the milk is expressed, the pressure decreases and milk production continues. You can express by hand or by using a pump, then bring the milk to the nursery for your baby.

While your baby is in the hospital and you are beginning to establish a milk supply, a pump will be most useful in stimulating and emptying your breasts. Pumps can be divided into two broad categories: those that are electric and those that are manually operated. Each type has certain advantages and disadvantages for mothers of premies. The electric pumps, such as the Egnell, the Medela, and the White River Electric Breast Pump, are excellent. They are comfortable and convenient to use. Many hospitals own electric pumps for the use of mothers while their babies are in the hospital. Ask a doctor or nurse if one is available for you and be sure to ask for a demonstration. Although a breast pump is easy to use once you know how, learning will be much easier if someone walks you through the steps the first time or two. These pumps are quite expensive, so not many people buy them for use at home. They are often available for rental, however, from drugstores and hospital supply stores throughout the United States. If your baby's physician prescribes the need for one, some insurance companies will reimburse you for its rental.

Manually operated pumps, such as the Kaneson (Marshall) pump and the Loyd-B-Pump (Lopuco, Inc.), are also convenient for expressing milk. Although you must create the suction by moving a cylinder back and forth on the Kaneson pump, the technique is easy to learn with a little practice. The Loyd-B-Pump will require somewhat more experience for you to learn to operate it smoothly because the suction and release phases are operated by different parts of the pump. These pumps are both relatively inexpensively priced, portable for use at home, hospital, or work, and easy to clean. They can be purchased through the respective companies or designated local outlets. Other suitable electric and manually operated pumps are available. New ones are frequently introduced. Check with your doctors, nurses, or local chapter of La Leche League for more information.

The one pump that is not acceptable is the manual one, sometimes called the bicycle horn, in which suction is created by your squeezing a bulb at the end. Bacteria are likely to infest the bulb, which cannot be adequately cleaned.

Collecting and Storing Breastmilk

Regardless of which pump you choose, it is essential that you keep it clean by sterilizing all pump parts and devices in which you collect the milk at least twice a day. You can do this by soaking them in boiling water or washing them in your dishwasher. Again, ask the nurses for information about the procedures they recommend for collecting and storing your milk. If you do not feed it to your baby immediately, you must be sure it is refrigerated or stored until he needs it.

The National Capital Lactation Center offers the following guidelines for storing breastmilk:

• Fresh breastmilk should be refrigerated and then used within twenty-four hours.

• Breastmilk may be frozen in the freezer compartment of your refrigerator for two weeks. If you have a separate freezer which cools to 0° F (or if your freezer compartment maintains this temperature), you may store your milk for six months.

• Put the date on the stored milk and use the oldest milk first.

Do not heat frozen or cooled breastmilk in boiling water. To thaw, put it under cool running water, gradually increasing the temperature of the water. You should not refreeze this milk.

Pumping and the Let-Down Response

Some mothers report that they rarely have a let-down response while using a machine. One mother told us her milk let down only twice while she was using an electric pump. The first time was when her husband appeared during her pumping session with the first pictures of their nine-day-old son. Her milk suddenly flowed, and she obtained twice as much as usual. The only other time she had a let-down response was the day before her son was coming home, when his crib had just been delivered and she tried expressing milk sitting in his soon-to-be-occupied room.

Barbara Happ, the former director of the National Capital Lactation Center at the Georgetown University Hospital, suggested two ways to encourage a let-down while you're pumping. When you pump in the morning, call the nursery to find out how your baby's night was. Hearing about him may be enough to trigger your response. Also, bring home some personal clothing or blankets that have touched or wrapped your baby. Smelling or feeling these while you pump will call all your senses into play and increase the chance of your having a let-down response.

Two neonatal nurses, Diana Stewart and Carol Gaiser, have written that "a strong emotional component as well as relaxation are the keys to the let-down" (p. 51). Knowing that relaxing can be very difficult for mothers who are worried about their hospitalized babies, these nurses have suggested a number of procedures to enhance milk production and foster your let-down response. Many of these are described in Chapter 2.

How Often to Express Milk

Although there is some difference of opinion, the experts generally agree that the first times you use an electric pump, two to five minutes on each breast are enough. You should gradually increase this time over the first three or four days until your breasts are emptied. Fifteen or twenty minutes on each breast should be all that is necessary. You should try to empty your breasts every three to four hours during the day to maintain your milk supply until your baby can nurse.

While your baby is in the hospital, you won't have to get up at night to express milk unless you feel more comfortable doing so. One mother said that she made the task more enjoyable by fixing up a cozy corner of her bedroom with a rocking chair next to the electric pump. She put all the congratulatory cards and telegrams on the wall and flowers on a table. Treating herself to a feminine nightgown and taping her baby's pictures on the pump made her feel more motherly, and she even got a better let-down response.

About a week before your baby comes home, you should start pumping once each night to build up a twenty-four-hour milk supply.

Feelings about Pumping

In our culture, because breasts are usually kept covered and rarely touched except in sexual play, the thought of expressing milk may make you feel uncomfortable at first. One woman probably voiced the views of many when she said that "being attached to a milking machine made me feel like I was part of a modern dairy." Once you become familiar with the idea of pumping, however, and once you master the technique and actually obtain milk for your baby, your uneasiness will probably diminish. Satisfying your baby's needs can become a source of great fulfillment for you.

One mother reported that after her daughter's birth, she told a nurse about her concerns about breastfeeding a premie. The nurse reassured her that she could, if she used a pump to build up her milk supply. Becoming comfortable using the electric pump was difficult: "I couldn't find a good position to sit in while trying to pump. My stitches were sore, and I had trouble sitting up in bed, leaning forward with my legs out. At first my brains were in a jumble. Just when I needed to think, I couldn't figure anything out. It was so demoralizing—being attached to that pump while the woman next to me was nursing a baby."

The first time this mother pumped, she got only a few drops of colostrum. "It didn't even cover the bottom of the little four-ounce bottle." By the third day, however, she was getting enough each session to fill about half an inch of the bottle. She had increased her pumping from about two to ten minutes per breast. She found it gratifying to see the increasing amount of milk she produced.

Expressing milk does take a lot of time and energy, but it is essential if you wish to nurse your baby when he is ready. In fact, if you want to nurse, maintaining your milk supply is one of your most important jobs while your baby is hospitalized.

Most mothers viewed pumping as a means to an end. One said, "All I wanted to do was put my milk in her. I figured I would express milk as long as I could and keep trying to get her to nurse." Another felt expressing milk for her baby gave them a physical link to each other. She felt satisfaction in the act of pumping because it was something she could do for her son. Other mothers said they enjoyed seeing the milk their bodies were making. Because they were pumping, they knew they could produce milk. They knew what it looked like. They knew how it came out. They were fascinated by all the tiny, separate streams of milk shooting from their nipples. One mother expressed her amazement at how different it was from milk dripping out of the hole in an artificial nipple. Many described the feelings of confidence they gained by seeing the milk they produced.

Putting Your Baby to Breast

If you are like most mothers who are expressing milk for their premature infants, you probably dream of holding your baby snugly in your arms for nursing. Yet when your moment finally arrives, you are likely to feel apprehensive. Not only do mothers feel nervous about a skill they've never practiced, but many also worry about how their babies will respond. Since mothers of premies often feel they can do little for their babies, nursing takes on added significance. Mothers want it to work so much that they feel very vulnerable. One woman said, "I wondered if he'd know me or think I was just another nurse." Several different mothers told us independently, "When my baby turned away from my breast, I felt that he didn't like me."

Try to remind yourself that nursing is a skill that takes practice to be mastered—for both you and your baby. Nursing is learned by nursing. Although your baby may be accustomed to the taste of your milk because you've been expressing it for him, he's not used to the taste, shape, or texture of your nipple. At first he does not know that the milk he likes has any association with the breast offered to him. He must learn this association through repeated experiences. A few babies will suck right away. If they get milk, they are on their way to learning the mother-breast-milk connection. If they don't get milk, they will need more chances to begin making the connections. When you can relax and follow your baby's initiatives without a deadline in mind for when "real nursing" should begin, the early experiences together can be enjoyed more readily.

One mother said that her baby, Aaron, did not nurse until a month after she took him home. At every feeding, Lucy Moore would offer Aaron her breast. He would turn away, thrash, get red, and refuse to nurse. Then she would give him expressed milk from a bottle and finally empty her breasts with a pump. She said she felt as though she was giving three feedings for each one. Suddenly, after a month at home, he started latching on and nursing. She said she managed to persist in trying for so long because a couple of times, when he just barely woke to eat in the middle of the night, he would nurse as though he'd always done it. "I knew he could do it, so I just kept trying." Lucy went on to nurse Aaron for eleven months.

The first time you put your baby to breast, it doesn't matter if he nurses. He really needs to explore. He needs the chance to smell, lick, touch, and taste the warm, soft skin of your breast and body. He needs to experience the pleasure of being cuddled and held skin-to-skin. Sucking is not the only, or even the primary, goal. His feeling relaxed, secure, and comfortable is what is crucial. The sucking and nursing will come in time. And if they don't, the snug physical contact you offer your child is invaluable to both of you.

Encouraging Nursing

You can help your baby be most comfortable while nursing by holding him on his side facing your breast. In this position he will not have to keep his head turned while actively grasping your nipple, sucking, and swallowing. If two pillows are placed on your lap, one under the baby and one behind his back, you can rest your arm on the pillow behind his back, cupping his buttocks in your hand. The crook of your arm supports his head in this position. Your baby can swallow easily, and you have a free hand, which you can use to guide the nipple to his mouth, press the fullness of your breast away from his nose, or reach for something to drink for yourself.

If your baby needs encouragement to suck, you may be able to squeeze a few drops of warm milk from your breast to interest him in the familiar taste. If your breasts are very full, expressing some milk will also help to soften the area around the nipple so your baby can latch on more easily. To help him grasp the nipple and breast with his tiny mouth, you should squeeze your breast behind the areola to flatten it and make the tip more pronounced. One mother said that when her baby yawned, she put her breast in his mouth. "He was surprised but started sucking!"

Nipple Confusion

Sucking the mother's nipple involves a very different motion than sucking a bottle. To nurse from you, the baby must "milk" your breast, first by using his jaws to compress the milk sinuses around the nipple, then by sucking the ejected milk into his mouth. The baby's whole face, from his jaws to his temples, seems to be involved in this energetic activity. Getting milk from a bottle, on the other hand, primarily involves the baby's stopping the fast flow of milk by pressing the artificial nipple against the roof of his mouth.

Since premies usually suck from artificial nipples first, they must learn a whole new method when they encounter the breast. Some babies seem confused by these two methods; others don't. One mother recalls watching her three-day-old daughter seem to pause between breast and bottle as though to register the difference before shifting gears. Confusion may be reduced by asking the nursery personnel to use a Nuk, Platex, or Enfamil "Natural" nipple, which resembles the shape of a human nipple in the baby's mouth. Patience and practice will also help, but some babies never do adapt to the breast. If yours is one of these, you may find nursing attempts to be so frustrating that you want to stop. Sometimes it is best to do so, remembering that you can continue to be a responsive mother, offering warm, secure contact while bottle feeding, too.

Frustrations with the Hospital

Learning to breastfeed in an intensive care nursery can be a very difficult proposition. The overall atmosphere usually ranges from strictly business to emergency. The number of people is often overwhelming. The schedules seem ironclad, and the comfortable space is at a minimum. Even in units that support breastfeeding, the overriding medical concerns often make tangible help and information hard to find. So parents of premies often experience different difficulties with the hospital than do parents of full-term babies.

One mother told us she always felt she was imposing when she came in to nurse her baby. "The impression I got—although nobody ever said it—was that I wanted to breastfeed to satisfy my own needs. Some nurses seemed to feel, 'If you insist on giving her breastmilk, at least give it in a bottle.' There just didn't seem to be time to fit breastfeeding into their schedule." Another mother had a delightfully different experience. She said, "Whenever I said I would be in to feed Sean, I'd find a note on his isolette that said, 'Hi! Don't feed me at 6. My mom will be here!' "

Many parents have commented on the difficulty of finding a private or even a quiet place to nurse. Some hospitals have mothers sit in unoccupied classrooms or storage rooms. Often a sign "Mother Breastfeeding" is put on the door. Yet strangers may persist in coming in for a variety of reasons. One father described the room where his wife nursed their baby as Grand Central Station.

It was an extra nursery that was used to store extra isolettes. But the phone rang constantly, people were always coming in and out, and two times babies were circumcised right there while Jean was trying to

nurse. I had to laugh at the usual advice to create a relaxed atmosphere
for my wife. We got assertive enough to ask for a particular office that
was usually quiet. But if the office wasn't available when Jean wanted
to nurse, there was nothing we could do. Creating calm was beyond
our control. We just did our best to ignore the hectic surroundings,
knowing one day we would take Amanda home.

Some mothers said that when no room was free, a hospital
screen was placed around them right in the nursery.

That was awful. Once a new baby had just been brought in and was
being examined three feet from me. I was physically separated, but in
the middle of an emergency. It may have been worse because I
couldn't see. I just heard the noises of doctor's orders, hurrying feet,
and baby's cries. And there I was sniffing my little bottle of Syntocinon—trying to get a let-down.

Many parents say they do not know how they got through the
early period of daily hospital visits. Most remember it as a very
trying time. Yet they coped because they felt their babies were
getting excellent medical care. A few mothers remarked that they
were exhausted once the period was over. One couple, Steve and
Marilyn Coyne, said their openness with each other was what got
them through. They shared their worries and anger as well as their
delight about their baby's progress. "Steve was my friend," Marilyn
said, "my confidant, my reality. When I felt Diane would never
nurse, he just held my hand and said she would. When he got
depressed because she still needed oxygen, I reminded him she
needed less than she did two days before. Nobody else loved her
like we did."

Finally, after what may seem like, or actually be, a hundred
hospital visits, a thousand meals on the run, and a million hours of
pumping, the time will come when you can take your baby home.
He has grown to about four or five pounds; he can maintain his body
temperature; he has no more problems requiring hospitalization;
and he can suck well enough to be gaining weight. You finally

become the ones responsible for his care. After days or weeks of being the assistants, the promotion to chief caregivers can be awesome.

Weight Gain and Giving Supplements

Many mothers report that they feel as though they are on probation from the time of discharge until that first doctor's visit when they're told the baby's doing fine—and especially that he is gaining weight well. With a premature baby, the emphasis on gaining is paramount. This may be especially hard for you, the breast-feeding mother, because some babies take awhile after they come home to start nursing well. The explicit ground rule is usually that if your baby doesn't gain, you will have to increase supplements or stop nursing.

The related issues of weight gain and using supplements are ticklish ones. Clearly the baby's weight gain is a measure of the nourishment he is getting. Clearly he must gain weight to thrive. The issue that is less clear is how much he must gain on a daily basis since weight is likely to fluctuate rather than increase steadily. Ideally, your baby's doctor will wholeheartedly support your desire to breastfeed, and you will fully trust him or her. If this relationship has developed, you can lean on the doctor for support in the trying period before your baby starts gaining well.

Mothers who have gotten through this period and continued to nurse their babies have usually attempted either not to supplement breastfeeding with extra bottles once home or to discontinue the bottles as soon as possible. Mothers who nurse, pump, then supplement for each feeding often find the time and energy involved in this regimen too difficult to sustain. A number of mothers of premies who stopped nursing early did so for this reason. One mother said, "At one month I was still giving supplements and nursing. It was too hard to do both. I dropped out the night-time nursing first, then another, until he was totally weaned." Other mothers, however, continue nursing and supplementing for months, finding this a comfortable and satisfying arrangement. You don't have to fulfill all your baby's nutritional requirements in order to enjoy breastfeeding.

Developing a Nursing Pattern:
Knowing When Your Baby Is Hungry

After feeding your baby by the clock in the intensive care nursery, you may be concerned about how you will know when your baby is hungry once home. This can be a special issue with premies, who are often very quiet and sleepy the first weeks at home. One mother said, "The first time Michael cried was weeks after we took him home. He didn't move either. While I slept at night he would sleep on my chest. We did that for weeks; he'd never move." Another mother described her son's cry as "a squeak." One mother said she'd wondered, "If Beth doesn't cry, how will I know she's hungry? How will I wake up at night?"

But mothers do learn to pick up signals of hunger by watching their babies closely—sometimes with the help of a friend who has had children of her own. One mother whose baby never cried said she could not tell when Sarah was hungry in their first days home. She tried to feed her every three hours, as she had in the hospital, but it wasn't working. Sarah wouldn't suck. Feeling desperate, she called a friend who had had a lot of experience with babies. Together they watched Sarah and discovered that she sometimes moved her hand toward her mouth in "a vague sort of way." "Feed her now, she's hungry," the friend suggested. It worked. From then on, that vague movement was considered the signal that Sarah wanted to nurse. Her timetable was not regular. Sometimes she nursed every hour; other times she'd wait for two or three hours. "We pretty much stayed at home that first month—upstairs in my room a lot of the time. Nursing Sarah was what I did."

Another mother found that even though her baby didn't cry, she would usually nurse if offered the breast whenever she woke up.

Usually that was every three or four hours. If she was still sleeping after four hours, her mother would awaken and feed her.

The nerves that tell the baby he is hungry may still be immature in the premie. Thus your doctor may set maximum limits for the lengths of time between feedings. In the first days especially, frequent feedings will help to assure that your baby's hunger is being satisfied and that you are getting enough sucking stimulation to build up your milk supply. If your baby is unresponsive, sleepy, and/or tires easily, nursing him during alert periods may work best. Diapering him, unwrapping him slightly, or bathing him may help him to awaken. Rocking a baby gently back and forth, then bringing him to an upright position at the adult's shoulder, often helps him come to an alert state. Calling their names softly a few times also helps some babies become alert. If your baby falls asleep, he may be saying he's had enough food and stimulation for the time being.

Many mothers told us that life was better, although sometimes trying, once they brought their babies home. Since you can be together all the time, you can learn what will work best for you both. But it isn't always easy. A few mothers said that in the beginning nursing their babies was much harder than using the breast pump because their babies were too drowsy or refused to suck. On the other hand, once home, mothers finally felt that their babies were really theirs. The efforts to nurse, though not always easy, seemed worthwhile.

5

Adjustments in the Early Months: The Baby

It was easier when I said to myself, "Look, this is the way things are going to be for a while and we'll all be better off if we just admit it."

—A NEW MOTHER

MY GRANDMOTHER, Anne Marie Doris, was a private-duty nurse in New York City in the first half of this century. Occasionally an assignment would take her to a household with a newborn. It was Grandma's opinion that it took a full twelve months of your life to have a baby: nine months in the womb and three months outside. Developmentally, the growing baby has similar needs whether in or out of the uterus. After birth the newborn's system requires the same constant physical and nutritional support that pregnancy earlier provided. Grandma believed that mothers and fathers set themselves up for frustration and disappointment when they expect a newborn to coordinate its systems and adapt to life outside the uterus too quickly.

We don't make attempts to shorten a pregnancy. We allow it to require nine months of our lives. But we seem less able to allow a newborn's adjustment period to take its required time.

"How long will this go on?" The mother may be referring to her newborn's seemingly constant nursing, her baby's frequent waking during the night, the infant's demand to be held all the time, or the baby's lengthy fussy periods. I remember asking the same question, feeling overwhelmed and exhausted three weeks after the birth of our first child. I was told by an experienced father that things would be a lot better when my daughter was three months old. *Three months!?* Did he have any idea how far away that was? At that moment I didn't feel confident that our new family was going to make it through the weekend, never mind getting to the three-month mark.

Some parents *do* report happy adjustment right around three months; for others the improvement is more gradual and less marked. Dr. Ann Oakley, a sociologist and researcher from Great Britain, who has spent years interviewing new mothers, has found that most women report feeling more positive and less anxious at five months (p. 246). Regardless of the timing—three months or five months—this does not mean a return to your "normal" life. That's one of the problems: measuring today by yesterday's standards.

Yesterday no baby totally depended upon you or could successfully rearrange your lives. A baby *does* that. You could say you won't have it—you won't permit it. You might just as well say that because you have so much you want to do (read, work, sew, study), you are no longer going to permit yourself to require sleep each day. You can't change your nature or your chemistry, and you can't change the nature or chemistry of a baby.

Much of what you might like to be different about living with a baby involves just those things that "come with the territory." One experienced mother of three children told us that there were times when she wished nursing would be "nicer, easier, better." She paused, smiled, and then added, "Of course, there were times when I wished that babies were nicer, easier, better."

Much of what goes on in those first weeks and months happens because you are becoming a mother, and you, your baby, and your husband are becoming a family. Breastfeeding adds a dimension to almost every aspect of your new role. In this and other chapters, we've chosen to discuss some issues that may appear at first to be unrelated to breastfeeding. Many of these, such as a baby's crying, schedules, and sleeping patterns, may seem to be general child care topics. It's our conviction, however, that breastfeeding cannot be separated from the other aspects of parenting and can be best discussed in light of the wide range of parenting activities. We believe that all of these child care considerations are affected by, or have an impact on, a mother's experience of nursing.

We interviewed several nursing mothers whose babies were under three months of age. It seems that two aspects of the newborn's behavior are most likely to concern, confuse, and exhaust the new parents—and to lead a woman to question her breastfeeding. These two issues are (1) a baby's fussing and (2) a baby's disorganized periods of wakefulness.

Fussy Times

In many homes new parents can spend the evening hours as they please. Their infant is fed and dry and snuggled in a soft, pastel sleeper and warm blanket, breathing serenely in his bassinet or crib. The parents have a chance to talk, shower, read the paper, or watch television without interruption and generally to enjoy their new sense of parenthood together. Perhaps this is how your nightlife begins. If so, congratulations! For who knows what reason, you have been blessed with an infant who uses the evening hours for sleeping. (This is what most of us *thought* babies did automatically.)

For many other new parents, the evening hours present a less tranquil scene. The new dad arrives home after a full day's work and commuter traffic to find both mother and infant in tears. The baby is having his "fussy time," and he is handed to his father, so that mother may do one of the things she's been trying to accomplish for the last hour: go to the bathroom, start dinner, get dressed, or have a shower.

Dinner is managed somehow. Mother nurses the baby at the table. Both parents are grateful that their newborn has calmed down and is willing to nurse. Other evenings one parent eats while the other walks the baby; then they exchange activities.

The infant may doze off once or twice during the evening before seriously going to sleep. And this dozing is generally accomplished only as the result of one parent walking, rocking, or nursing the baby. Both parents get to watch Johnny Carson's "Tonight Show" in its entirety (something to which neither adult ever aspired) before getting the baby seriously to sleep.

The parents have no trouble going to sleep at 2 A.M. A few quick thoughts simultaneously skitter through the mother's mind before she slips off into much needed sleep: Maybe I can get three hours straight before the baby wakes to nurse. Any night now he'll probably sleep right through the whole night. We're never going to survive this.

Why is he so fretful?

You can't be sure. Often, one of the problems for a new breastfeeding mother is her readiness to assume that her baby's fussing is related to the quantity or quality of her milk. In fact, there are many other possible explanations. Remember what we said earlier: It may take three months (and perhaps more) for your newborn to adjust to life outside the womb. These first months can be trying and disconcerting for your infant, who can do very little to comfort himself. Perhaps the two most effective activities in his repertoire are sucking and crying. The sucking guarantees that he can get food into his mouth. It also helps the baby to calm himself. The crying is *meant* to guarantee that someone will help him in his distress, which may be related to hunger, temperature change, pain, loneliness, need for body contact, or need for movement.

Most of these sources of distress were absent in your womb. Your baby's needs were marvelously (and almost effortlessly, on your part) taken care of during the nine months of pregnancy. The placenta provided nutrition so that your unborn baby never felt hunger. He felt no discomfort from diaper rash or abrupt changes in temperature. He was guaranteed the soothing, rhythmic sounds of your heart beating and your blood pumping. His whole life in your uterus provided him with gentle movement in the amniotic fluid and regular rocking whenever you moved. He was enclosed, held truly close inside your body. Now he's out with you, and the environment he had known until birth is gone. Now you and your husband need to respond actively to your infant's needs. Does it really matter that you don't know why he's fussy?

Your newborn needs time to adjust to this new environment. Within his new loving and supportive surroundings, he can learn that his requests, even his demands, will be honored. Someone will respond to his frightening hunger—not in an hour for the sake of a schedule but *now* for the sake of a hungry baby. He will gain confidence in his world when he learns that he can count on you to respond to his biological and emotional needs for closeness, for body contact, for soothing motion.

If your baby does have fussy periods, which often occur in the evening, take solace. This will not go on forever. But it's impossible for anyone to predict how long the fussy periods will plague you and your baby. Some babies persist in this behavior (to some degree) for several weeks or even months; others manage to calm down in one or two weeks. Some newborns have fussy times that can last for three hours; others are fretful for just an hour. Some will calm down if they are simply held; others require the motion of walking or rocking. One of our children was most relaxed when his father simultaneously rocked and jiggled him, creating a motion similar to that of a car driving on a rocky country road.

If you feel that some of your baby's irritability might be caused by your tenseness, you might want to see if you can learn to relax a little. This may not be easy, particularly when there are other demands on you, such as a job, phone calls, and other children. One way to become more relaxed with your baby is to get to know him better.

In the beginning, taking care of the baby often presents itself as a job, a series of activities to be accomplished: bathe, nurse, change, dress warmly, get him to sleep. But through these everyday activities, you will discover your baby's uniqueness and allow him to discover yours. If these "chores" are always hurried, opportunities are being missed for gentle handling, soft conversation, smiling, observing, and lingering. Lingering with your baby is not "wasting time." For some new mothers, who have always worked efficiently at home or on the job, it may *seem* to be, and the habit of "getting the job done" can be a difficult one to break.

The drive to be efficient can present a special problem for breastfeeding mothers. Some babies *do* get right down to the business of feeding, but others do not. A young mother of a five-week-old daughter found her baby's style of nursing most exasperating. Nancy Cohen told us, "I want to say to her: 'If you want to eat, then eat. If you're not going to, then let's stop.'" Nancy explained that she had no idea beforehand that a baby could suck and then stop, suck and then stop. She found this a very inefficient method of getting food into her baby.

Another mother expressed frustration at the time required for each feeding. Cathy Stanford told us, "When the books said I should nurse ten minutes on each side, I thought I'd be finished in twenty minutes. It can really be frustrating when you want the baby to get down to business and he wants to lounge around in the middle of a feeding. It can take us twenty to twenty-five minutes to get ten minutes of sucking."

This mother's experience is not uncommon. With newborns, nursings can be very time-consuming. This usually changes (except during occasional growth spurts) as your baby gets older. Meanwhile, other things are happening during these early feedings that are important to your infant's overall development. Your baby is beginning to memorize your face. He is beginning to know the feel of your arms, the smell and touch of your skin. He is beginning to learn about his own abilities. He can latch on and suck and get milk to swallow. He can let go. He has some control.

Although some slowing down is, therefore, productive in the

mother-baby relationship, you will not spend each feeding in this quiet, reflective fashion. Running a household and coping with distractions from a job, friends, and other family members will demand your attention. Thus in the course of establishing breastfeeding, there are likely to be quick or agitated feedings, as well as unhurried and satisfying ones. Managing to balance these experiences—welcoming the calm opportunities and accepting the less-than-perfect ones—is part of the adjustment process.

Calming a Fussy Baby

Your baby may be irritable for any one or a combination of reasons. Certainly, if he hasn't nursed in the last hour and a half, or if he fell asleep midway through a nursing forty-five minutes ago, you should offer him the breast again. He may be hungry. You may want him to go three or four hours between feedings like a good bottle-fed baby, but your baby is growing on breastmilk. The "rules" are different because your milk is different (see Chapter 1).

Whether or not he's hungry, you may want to let him nurse, because some babies need extra sucking and are calmed by it. But as good as breastmilk and nursing are, they won't fix everything. Your fussy infant may benefit from one or more other interventions.

YOUR DIET.   Your baby's fussiness could be a reaction to some food in your diet. What you eat will be passed on to your baby through your milk. Some women can eat anything with no apparent reaction in their babies. Other mothers have told us that when they cut out or cut down on a particular substance, their babies' fussiness subsided.

If you have allergies in your family, your baby is a candidate for allergies. The most common allergen in babies is cow's milk. If you are consuming a considerable amount of dairy products—milk, cheese, ice cream, yogurt—you may be passing on to your infant incompletely metabolized foreign proteins in your milk to which the baby reacts. According to JoAnne Scott, a certified lactation consultant in Annandale, Virginia,

Other things to watch out for in your diet are foods which cause *you* discomfort: foods which give you gas, indigestion, heartburn, or to which you may have been allergic at some point in your life, even though you think you have outgrown the allergy. Any food you craved during pregnancy and ate in large quantities could have sensitized the baby in utero. Any food you are very fond of and miss if it is absent from your diet for even one day is another likely candidate. We can be addicted to foods to which we are allergic. Other substances which sometimes bother totally breastfed babies are the colorings and flavorings in baby vitamins, fluoride drops, and the stool-softeners commonly found in the mother's prenatal vitamins.

It is commonly believed that nursing mothers should avoid onions and spices. If you customarily consume highly spiced foods, you can probably continue to do so. Spices and onions flavor your milk, but seldom bother the baby. Latin, Greek, Indian, and Oriental women who are accustomed to highly spiced diets go right on and nurse their babies. However, if you eat the traditional bland American diet and then go out for a Mexican dinner when your baby is several months old, he may reject your milk the next day. Onions and spices will flavor your milk. If your baby is accustomed to such flavors from the beginning, they will be normal for him. But if they are only occasional, they may startle him (Personal communication).

CLOSENESS.   Since babies often enjoy being held and cradled, many parents use a fabric baby carrier that keeps the baby close to your chest but frees your hands. With the baby strapped to your chest or to your husband's chest, you may be able to eat dinner with two hands and without the background music of an unhappy baby.

MOTION.   Sometimes the carrier isn't enough. It's often necessary to stand and sway back and forth. It's not the conventional dining or relaxing posture, but it can be done effectively. One couple we met, both of whom were lawyers, had been used to enjoying relaxed, well-planned dinners with a bottle of wine and candles. "Things are dramatically different now," Ellen Horst said. "I'm home all day, but there is less time to cook and less time to eat. Dinners are quicker and less fancy. If we're lucky, Justin will allow one of us to push him back and forth in the umbrella stroller—I can manage that with my feet now—while we eat a hurried meal. There are times when only one of us is seated at the table. The other one is walking, jiggling, or dancing with Justin."

Another couple discovered that riding in a car was magic for calming their baby. Several times a week, once dad arrived home, they would all get in the car and run errands. This allowed the grown-ups time for conversation and provided the baby with the sensations that relaxed her. Whether they picked up clothes at the cleaners or a pizza for dinner, these short outings were good for all three of them.

Many of the mothers we spoke to had used wind-up swings or cradles to get a break from rocking or carrying their babies. Some babies seem to enjoy the swings; others become more agitated. Keep in mind that a wind-up swing might *not* do the trick, could be expensive, will take up a lot of room, and is often needed or useful for only a matter of weeks. We strongly recommend that you first try to borrow one, if you're interested in one.

SOUND.   Most of the treatments for a fussy baby involve body contact, motion, or both. Another possibility is sound. Some infants can be soothed by a rhythmic, repeated lullaby or the gentle tones of a music box. Others prefer the monotonous ticking of a wind-up alarm clock. And a few find real peace in the sounds of the dishwasher or vacuum cleaner. Marylou Ostengo explained her "discovery" to us.

> One day I felt as though I was really being pushed over the edge. I was convinced that what Tommy needed was sleep. He wouldn't nurse anymore and I had been walking or rocking him for hours. I finally decided I had to accomplish something and distract myself from Tommy. I took out the vacuum cleaner, positioned Tommy over my shoulder, and turned on the machine. It was as if someone had injected Valium into his veins. He went limp, whimpered once or twice, and was out! I couldn't believe what I had discovered! Sometimes it would be one or two in the morning when we would have to resort to vacuuming Tommy to sleep. It was summer and our windows were

open. I suppose our neighbors wondered about my compulsive cleaning habits!

Some newborns do seem to need help in blocking out the bombardment of stimuli around them. The vacuum cleaner noise, in Tommy's case, blocked out all other information from his environment and freed him to sleep. The strength of the noise might also have provided some comforting vibration. If the vacuum cleaner seems a bit extreme, you might park your baby near the automatic dishwasher when you turn it on. Sometimes even the sound of running water soothes a baby. And one woman found success when she used her sewing machine and draped her baby across her knees.

RESPONDING TO CRYING. Finally, what about letting your baby "cry it out" when he is fretful? Some infants need a little crying time before drifting off to sleep. A *little* crying time. Letting the baby cry until he falls asleep, if that means an hour or more of crying, seems most inhumane. Listen to your baby. Is the crying subsiding or getting more frantic? Give him ten or fifteen minutes. If he doesn't seem to be crying himself to sleep, but rather crying himself into a frenzy, then go to him. Some babies can be successfully nursed or rocked to sleep after a ten-minute cry. Some infants, if allowed to cry too long, work themselves into such a frantic state that you must work even harder to sooth them. As you get to know your baby and discover his style, you probably will develop effective ways to help him settle down.

As we listened to couples discuss crying babies, it became clear that many of them share one big worry: If we keep responding to his crying, we'll be letting him *manipulate* us. It's not surprising that this fear exists. A look through some parenting magazines and books suggests that this fear is fostered by many experts: "Above all, do *not* let yourself be manipulated by a baby!"

Let's take another look at this issue.

A baby is *supposed* to learn to manipulate his environment. If a baby is to grow into a young child who trusts you and much of his small world, if he is to feel safe and secure, he must learn early on that his surroundings are, in fact, trustworthy. He learns that he can count on you because you respond to him. Even if you can't always soothe him, you are giving him an important message by staying with him. You won't always be able to fix things for your child, but offering your presence may be very important.

Your baby cries, you respond. In fact, you are teaching your baby that his attempts at *communication* are working. As limited and dependent and immature as he is, he has *one* ability by which he can communicate his needs and desires—*if* someone will listen. Some researchers have studied babies whose mothers respond to their cries "promptly and warmly." The results of this study indicate that by the end of the first year, these babies cry less than babies who are ignored or restricted or scolded.

Nightlife

> *Wee Willie Winkie runs through the town*
> *Upstairs and downstairs in his nightgown*
> *Rapping at the windows, crying through the locks*
> *"Are the babies all in bed? For now it's eight o'clock."*

Is your baby sleeping through the night yet? That's the big question. One mother we spoke to wanted to know if midnight to 5 A.M. could qualify as "through the night." "I just need to be able to tell people that she's sleeping through," Audrey Gibbs said. "I'm not sure it matters so much to me, but it's one of the first questions people ask."

If you must explain that your baby wakes once, twice, or three times a night, your response often just hangs there in the air in front of you. Sometimes people don't know what to say to you. Your questioner may be privately appalled at such uncivilized routines, or amazed that you can function so well, or embarrassed that he has learned something so revealing about your ability to be a mother. Your questioner may even offer some advice as to how to "cure" your child of this habit. All this may occur, unless your answer is heard by sympathetic parents who've been there—and who remember the journey.

Some babies manage to sleep long stretches at night at an early age. Many do not. This may have as much to do with their innate temperaments as anything else. It may also have something to do with normal variations in individual development, in the same way that some babies walk at ten months and others at fourteen months. Often a major concern for the breastfeeding mother revolves around a suspicion that, if she gives up breastfeeding and offers formula instead, her baby will sleep through the night. Another concern is that, if the baby is totally breastfed, nighttime feedings require the mother's presence and this can mean a serious lack of sleep for her. In this chapter we will address these issues.

A common nighttime pattern for a newborn is to wake two, three, or more times a night, nurse easily, but then be difficult to get back to sleep. Susan Harrison, whose son exhibited this pattern, explained her frustration: "I felt so out of control. John and I rocked him and walked him and jiggled him. What was wrong? Why couldn't I fix it? I started thinking that they shouldn't have let us take him home till we knew what to do with him. I cried a lot. I felt helpless."

Susan claimed that she was almost obsessed with the issue of sleeping through the night. She had an "incredible craving" for a night's sleep, but she understood that, in the early weeks, nighttime nursings were valuable for building up her milk supply. It wasn't even the nursing she found difficult: "It was the crying. It drove me almost to distraction. The nursing took maybe twenty minutes, but getting Jason back to sleep could take another thirty minutes or an hour. And this would happen maybe three times a night. It got so that at the beginning of a feeding I'd get tense, wondering how long it would be before I'd get to go back to sleep."

Susan's husband convinced her to express some of her own milk during the days so that one night he could feed Jason and Susan could sleep. This provided immeasurable relief for Susan, who slept in the spare bedroom that night. Only a few nights later, Jason slept a full six hours, from 12:30 A.M. to 6:30 A.M. He was about seven weeks old.

When we talked to Susan, Jason was three months old and was still sleeping an uninterrupted six-hour stretch at night. She told us, "When Jason was finally on some kind of predictable schedule— even though it was only predictable at night—that was the real turn-around. I relaxed a bit and really started to enjoy him."

Another common pattern is the infant who sleeps well in the first couple of weeks after birth but then begins to be wakeful and fretful at night. Karen Lambert's baby, Jessica, though generally irritable in the evening, was able to settle down to sleep at about ten in the evening. During the night she nursed efficiently about every two hours and went back to sleep effortlessly until she was two weeks old.

Then things changed. Jessica would be put to bed at ten and would be crying and fussing before eleven. Karen said, "I was in and out of bed all the time, because she just wasn't able to calm down and sleep. It could go on till two or three in the morning. I started to realize there was no point in fighting this."

Karen changed *her* routine. Her husband went to bed in the bedroom. Karen got ready for bed, but she and Jessica headed for the living room. Karen nursed her baby every two hours and often walked around the room with Jessica on her shoulder. In addition to the walking routine, Karen also tried to help Jessica burp or pass gas. Sometimes she sat and draped the baby over her knees and rubbed Jessica's back. Sometimes she massaged her body. "As long as I held her close, we seemed to be okay. Sometimes, after she calmed down, I'd prop myself on the couch and sleep with her on my chest. If I tried to put her down, within seconds she'd startle awake and the whole thing could start again."

For a time during those early weeks, Karen tried to continue "business as usual" for her family.

I wanted everything to be nice for everyone. I wanted to look good when Jack came home from work, so I found myself tensing up if I hadn't even had time to comb my hair. I wanted us to have calm, nutritious dinners . . . on time. I wanted my two-year-old to feel as though I still belonged to him, so I insisted on reading him his bedtime stories. And this was all happening as Jessica was beginning to work herself into her fussy time. One night I burned the entire chicken and the peas and carrots. So much for nutritious dinners! I just wept.

Karen admitted she *couldn't* do everything. Routines changed. Dinners for the grown-ups were later, after two-year-old Brian had had his story (often read by dad) and had gone to sleep. After a particularly bad night, Karen would sometimes go to bed when Jack came home at six. She would get up at eight to nurse Jessica and then would go back to bed until ten, when she would take over for the rest of the night. Karen also learned to nap during the children's naps in the afternoon. "It was easier when I said to myself, 'Look, this is the way things are going to be for a while and we'll all be better off if we just admit it.' I had to stop thinking I could fix everything. I had to remind myself that what I was doing for Jessica during the night was valuable."

By the time Jessica was three months old, she was still somewhat fussy during the evening but was asleep by ten and generally slept until three. She nursed quickly and quietly and went back to sleep easily.

Why Are Some Babies So Wakeful at Night?

SLEEP REQUIREMENTS.   A glance at some books about babies would suggest that an infant's routine involves a morning nap, an afternoon nap, and a night of ten or twelve hours of sleep. In real life, babies vary considerably in their needs for sleep. *Some infants may require as much as eighteen to twenty hours a day; others need as little as ten hours.* Because parents of a newborn are likely to be concerned about whether their baby is normal—is he really okay?—this wide variation can cause some worry. If baby sleeps a lot, parents may worry that their child is too lethargic, not alert. If a child only catnaps during the day and sleeps little at night, parents may worry that their baby is too nervous, high-strung.

In either case, the eventual question regarding babies who are extreme in their sleeping habits is "Can this be healthy for him?" Be assured that an infant does not make plans to stay up if he truly needs to sleep, nor does he decide to sleep when he has no need for sleep. You or I or any given three-year-old may behave in such a fashion, but a newborn is genuine in his needs for such things as food and sleep. Trust him.

If you have a baby who needs and enjoys lots of sleep, you should do three things: (1) appreciate the time this allows for you; (2) play with, hold, talk, and sing to your baby when he's awake; and (3) make sure that, in the early weeks, you are nursing him seven to eleven times in each twenty-four-hour period.

If you have a baby who requires very little sleep, you need to realize four things: (1) his style of sleeping is not a problem for him, though it may be a problem for you; (2) you may need to nap whenever the baby does in order to get *your* required sleep; (3) although this child may never require *much* sleep, as he grows and becomes more active, it is likely that he will sleep more than he does now; and (4) there are *many* babies like yours and *many* mothers who were surprised—maybe shocked—to find that newborns don't necessarily sleep all the time.

FEEDING REQUIREMENTS. Nighttime feedings generally play an important part in establishing and maintaining a mother's milk supply. In the early months, some babies nurse about every one and a half to three hours both day and night. Other infants, at least in the beginning, nurse less frequently during the day and more frequently during the night. This may be because the baby is more relaxed and less distracted during nighttime feedings; it may also be that the mother is more relaxed and less distracted and therefore her let-down reflex is more easily triggered. After a few weeks of breast-feeding, as the mother's let-down reflex becomes more conditioned, and as the baby becomes more capable of shutting out some distractions on his own, this pattern of frequent night feedings may change. Finally, there are babies who, happily for their parents, choose to sleep five or six or more hours at a stretch during the night. Since such a baby still requires the same amount of food as if he were not sleeping those hours, he needs to make up for lost time. As a result, some of his early morning or daytime feedings may be only one hour apart.

Because of the composition of human mother's milk, low in protein and low in fat (discussed in Chapter 1), it is logical that some nighttime feedings are necessary. It is very likely that your waking baby has digested your milk and is, in fact, hungry. According to Dr. Derrick B. Jelliffe, coauthor of *Human Milk in the Modern World,* breastfeeding at night is considered usual and normal in traditional cultures. Even in the United States, before the turn of the century and the gradual decline in breastfeeding, nighttime nursings were considered routine. Although some babies manage to sleep for longer periods at night, it is likely that the universal expectation of "sleeping through" was fostered as a result of formula feeding.

FORMULA OR CEREAL. If you are living with a baby who wakes frequently at night, you may have thought of giving him formula or even cereal for the bedtime feeding.

When he was two weeks old, we started feeding him cereal at bedtime and that's when he started sleeping right through!

Why don't you give her some formula for the last feeding and see if that works?

Certainly, filling up the baby with formula or cereal could mean he won't wake with hunger in two or three hours. Before you resort to such an option, however, you should have more information.

• Formula *will* stay in your baby's tummy longer because it is higher in protein and fat. By the same token, it is less digestible than breastmilk. This means that some babies will have intestinal disturbances as their immature digestive systems try to deal with the formula. As a result, your baby may not be comfortable and may not sleep any better or any longer. (Some babies do not have any apparent difficulties with formula, especially if they are not given cow's milk formulas.)

• Some babies who are totally breastfed begin to sleep through in the early weeks of life. Other children do not sleep through the night for years. It may be a matter of temperament, style, or maturation. Such children, even when they're eating cheeseburgers for dinner, still wake once or twice a night. When such a child is an infant, he wakes and cries for you. Once he is awake, he may notice he is also hungry. Thus he may be satisfied by nursing. Even if he is not hungry, nursing may soothe him back to sleep.

• It's not a good idea to begin your baby on solids in the first months of his life. According to the Committee on Nutrition of the American Academy of Pediatrics (1980) it wasn't until about 1920 that infants under one year of age were offered solids. Breastmilk or cow's milk formulas supplied all or most of the nutrition requirements for that first year of life. In the decades after 1920, the baby food industry grew, and solid foods were offered to babies earlier and earlier, sometimes within the first ten or fourteen days of life. Certainly, the advertising and promotion campaigns launched by baby food companies must have had something to do with the earlier use of solids. In addition, according to the report of the Committee on Nutrition, "Some of the reasons for earlier introduction of solid foods were the desire of mothers to see their infants gain weight rapidly, the ready availability of convenient forms of solid foods, and *the mistaken assumption that added solid foods help the infant to sleep through the night"* (*Pediatrics,* June 1980, p. 1178).

The current recommendation for introduction of solids is to wait until the baby is about six months old. Some authorities recommend waiting even longer, particularly if there is a history of serious allergies in your family or if the use of solid foods means a serious reduction in your baby's intake of breastmilk and therefore of the immunological protection provided by breastmilk.

COLIC. Many babies have regular fussy, colicky periods during the evening hours; other infants experience intestinal distress in the wee hours of the morning. These babies, then, are not simply wakeful; they can be miserable and difficult to soothe. If, as some authorities now think, colic means the baby is suffering gastrointestinal discomfort as the result of an immature digestive system, and immature nervous system, or both, offering formula would be a mistake. The only real cure for this physical immaturity is time.

One mother described her reaction to her one-month-old's fretful nights.

> I was so frustrated. One night, when nothing was working—Michael was still fussing and crying—I was so exasperated. By then, *I* was crying, too. I took him in my arms and said, "Why don't you go to sleep? *Why?*" I wondered if it was my fault. My diet? Should I cut out milk? Ice cream? Orange juice? Leafy green vegetables? Every book seemed to say something different. After a while I figured that what I had read about colic seemed to apply to Michael. And while I was very conscientious about eating carefully, I decided it was mostly a problem with his immature digestive system, and we'd just have to wait it out.

Many parents claim that by three months the colicky fussing begins to disappear. Nevertheless, "waiting it out" can be draining and seem endless. In this chapter we have offered some suggestions for calming a fussing baby. It's possible that, like many other mothers, you will discover your own combination of techniques that will be effective for you. It's also possible that nothing will work or work for very long. In either case, it's important for you and your husband to arrange to get as much sleep as you can *when* you can. It's also important to realize that this problem, which challenges your sanity and your sense of humor, is temporary and will diminish regardless of what you do.

GROWTH SPURTS. With some babies, sleeping through the night is an on-again, off-again thing. There are times when the baby will go five, six, or seven hours at a stretch. One week later, the same baby wakes to nurse every two hours. This infant may be experiencing a growth spurt. These commonly occur at ten to fourteen days, five to six weeks, three months, and six months. During these times, your baby is driven to nurse more frequently. His more frequent sucking will send the message to your brain to produce more milk. If allowed unlimited access to the breast, your baby can accomplish his task in two or three days. After each growth spurt, it is common for the baby to go back to his former routines. If the baby is not allowed to nurse frequently, it will take longer for your milk supply to build up to meet the new needs of your growing baby. Understanding the purpose of your baby's increased need to nurse may help you get through the demands of his frequent feedings, although you still may not feel exactly happy about it. One mother, talking about these growth spurts, told us that she felt less like a mother and more like a twenty-four-hour snack bar.

COPING WITH WAKEFUL NIGHTS.   Much of your ability to cope with your baby's wakeful nights will probably depend on your attitude. And your attitudes about nighttime sleeping may have to be reorganized. Most of us start with certain basic beliefs, which, as parents of infants tell us, just are *not* necessarily so:

- I require eight hours of sleep each night.
- I have a *right* to eight hours of sleep.
- If sleep is to be useful, it should be uninterrupted.

Similar to your baby, you have certain sleep habits and sleep requirements. The routines that develop around your baby's nighttime waking will have a lot to do with your feelings about sleep, schedules, your new role, your husband's role, and the place of the new baby in your lives. Some of your most strongly held opinions may change as your life as a mother develops. It's important to know that many of the alterations in your nighttime schedule will not be as dramatic after the first several weeks. Many of the changes you have to make will be only temporary. And keep in mind that even though you may be *willing* to live your life in topsy-turvy fashion for a while, that doesn't mean you are going to *like* it!

One twenty-nine-year-old mother of a newborn explained that as she walked her son back and forth in the bedroom between midnight and 3:30 A.M., she spent half the time resenting her crying, unhappy baby, thinking life was awfully unfair. The other half of the time, she felt a part of humanity, vital in her role as a capable, giving mother, and convinced that she was making an investment in her son's emotional well-being.

Rosemary Duran, the mother of a two-and-a-half-month-old daughter, spoke about similar feelings of ambivalence:

> I keep telling myself that I really like this little baby, and I'm liking her more and more, but I just wish she didn't need me so much, especially at night. I have a fantasy which I play out over and over again in my head. I look at the clock while I'm nursing the baby and then turn to my husband and say, "Oh, it's eight o'clock. I guess I'll put Kathryn to bed now." And, in my fantasy, it works. I put her in her crib and she sleeps.
>
> In real life, she goes to bed in our bed at 2 A.M. I guess we're all getting used to it. It's not such a big deal as it was that first month. In some ways I like her being close to us. But I sure would like that baby who goes to bed at eight o'clock!

Parents who spend time trying to get their babies to sleep during those early morning hours resort to a variety of activities. In addition to the suggestions mentioned earlier for dealing with a fussy baby, here are some other ideas that might help you to calm the baby and get him to sleep or perhaps maintain your own sanity while the baby is wakeful. Keep in mind that these long nights are only *temporary.* As your infant matures and becomes more capable in this world outside the uterus, life will become more manageable and predictable.

• Place the baby in a baby carrier on your chest and free yourself to do some additional activity (regardless of the unconventional hour for such activity). Remember, it may also be necessary to sway back and forth. Some parents feel better if they are doing two things at once: calming the baby *and* baking or reading or folding laundry or needlepointing or dusting.

• If the baby falls asleep in the carrier, get comfortable in a recliner or in your bed or on the couch and go to sleep yourself with the baby snuggled on your chest, secure within the carrier.

• One dad we spoke to was the primary caretaker of his new daughter. He stayed at home during the day when his wife was teaching school. In those early weeks, he regularly took his baby for a midnight car ride, after the mother had finished nursing. Once his daughter was soundly sleeping he could carry her into the house and place her in the bassinet.

• One mother, after failing to get her son to adapt to mom's preferred schedule, reorganized her own sleep routine. She decided she would pretend she was working the evening shift at a new job, and she considered 2 or 3 A.M. to be her own new "bedtime"; 11:00 A.M. became the time she got up. Although it was impossible to get the baby to sleep before 2 A.M., once he went to sleep he woke only twice for relaxed feedings and went back to sleep easily. This mother found herself more relaxed once she accepted the new routine. A radical change in schedule was possible for this woman because she had no other children and hadn't returned to a job.

• One couple, Sharon and Hank Shuba, formulated a plan whereby each adult could get a good night's sleep at least one night a week, usually during the weekend. Their bedroom, with the baby's cradle, was designated the "war room"; the guest bedroom was the "recovery room." If Sharon was on duty, she and baby spent the night in the war room, and Hank slept uninterrupted in the recovery room. If dad was on duty, it was Sharon's turn for the recovery room. Each time the baby woke for a feeding, Hank would bring him into the mother's bed. After Sharon nursed him, she was able to drift off to sleep, while father and son returned to the war room for walking and rocking and eventual sleeping.

• Since your infant is continually developing and maturing, his responses to your attempts to comfort him may change. What worked last month may no longer work. On the other hand, earlier measures that failed may now succeed. Whereas a few days ago your infant may have screamed inconsolably if you put him down in his crib to sleep after nursing him, now he may simply offer a slight protest or cry weakly for a few minutes and then go off to sleep. It's worth reconsidering earlier ideas from time to time.

• One mother told us that she felt less tense and tired if she did not know exactly how much sleep she was missing each night. Therefore, she chose not to look at the clock each time her baby woke her.

• Because exhaustion can be such a problem when babies are young, some parents decided to take their fussy or wakeful baby into bed with them. Many of these parents told us that they had not considered this option before they had their baby.

SLEEPING AROUND.   Babies have always slept with their mothers. In many families around the world they still do. It is only in the last century, in the Western world, that the custom of separate sleeping arrangements has become popular. That is certainly a very recent development when you consider that our species has been around for a couple of million years. Perhaps separate sleeping will prove to be nothing more than a fad in the history of mankind. Our culture may very well be "going through a phase."

When you consider the many needs of a baby—warmth, contact, readily available food, rhythmic sound, closeness, reassurance—allowing the baby to sleep with you can provide an easy way to satisfy these needs. Still, as logical as that may seem, the feeling persists that it is not right.

The question of whether to take your baby into your room or into your bed is probably best answered by the authorities who are most closely involved: you and your husband. If you look to outside authorities, you will find conflicting advice. Some psychiatrists will warn against it. Some child development experts and anthropologists will encourage it. In an issue of a popular magazine for parents, a pediatrician spoke out firmly against all but the most minimal nighttime contact. The same magazine ran a cover story seven months later which spent five pages discussing the positive aspects of children sleeping with their parents. What would be best for you and your child? Your decision should not be based solely on which magazine article you read or entirely on what your mother or pediatrician tells you. You must discover for yourselves what arrangement is workable and acceptable.

Several objections are often raised against sleeping with a baby. For example, you may be concerned about maintaining your sex life with a baby in your room or in your bed. Some parents handle this problem by making love in another room once the baby is asleep. For those whose baby may sleep first in his own room and join the parents only after waking during the night, the parents' own bed is available for the first part of the night. And for most new mothers and fathers, sex is not so easy nor so frequent during those first months after a new baby arrives, *regardless* of where that new baby is sleeping.

A frequent worry in the early months is that a parent will roll over on the baby and hurt or smother him. Lactation consultant JoAnne Scott addresses this concern:

> You are not unconscious when you are asleep—you are semiconscious. You don't roll on your baby any more than you roll off the side of your bed. You are very aware, at all times, of where your baby is.

> The widespread fear of "over-laying" a baby seems to stem from two sources: Sudden Infant Death Syndrome, which even today can be mis-diagnosed as smothering, and an apparently widespread practice of heroin abuse among 18th century English wet-nurses. When all babies slept in their parents' beds, SIDS was thought to be a result of overlaying. Now that most babies sleep in cribs, it is called "crib death." As long as you haven't taken such consciousness-altering substances as drugs or excessive alcohol, you won't roll on your baby. (Personal communication)

Another common objection to taking the baby into your bed is
the worry that, once you start it, you'll never be able to break the
child of the habit. Yet we don't seem to have these worries about
other aspects of infant care. For example, would you take seriously
the following advice? "Don't let your baby get used to diapers, or
you'll never break him of the habit" or "If you let your baby suck
on your breasts now, she'll always want to do that." Most of us
believe that when the time is right for both the child and the parent,
toilet training and weaning will occur. We may need the same faith
regarding sleeping patterns and sleeping arrangements.

Parents give several reasons for taking their babies into their
rooms or their beds. Most often the initial reason had a lot to do with
everyone's need for sleep. As one mother commented, "It isn't just
easier for the baby; it's easier for us, too." The bodily closeness
throughout the night seems to be beneficial for both mother and
infant. It may be that this nighttime closeness helps synchronize both
the mother's and the infant's sleep cycles, and, therefore, a mother
may be less often awakened from a deep sleep.

In addition, you can respond to your infant without disrupting
your sleep in a major way—there's no getting out of bed, going to
your baby's room, and sitting up to nurse. Also, because you are so
close and therefore able to hear him as he begins to wake, your baby
does not have to wake himself so thoroughly by crying loudly to get
your attention. A baby who needs to make only a few waking sounds
and movements will be more easily nursed back to sleep. Perhaps
by having your infant close by and deciding to be easily available to
him throughout the night, you may be able to get more sleep yourself and feel more relaxed both day and night.

In the final analysis, you need to discover the nighttime routine
that best suits you and your new family. Not all couples are comfortable with the family bed idea. It's an approach that is not widely
practiced in contemporary culture, but because so many couples told
us that they had eventually chosen this option, we wanted to present
it as one of the choices in nighttime parenting.

Caring for a newborn places enormous demands on your time,
ingenuity, and stamina. Most mothers would agree that the details

of living with a baby can be imagined beforehand, but the intensity of that experience cannot. The dilemmas that arise regarding the baby's nursing, crying, and sleeping are real and crucial only once there is a real baby. Becoming a mother requires on-the-job training. As is true with most new jobs, you are apt to have periods of confusion and some feelings of inadequacy.

As the weeks and months pass, important changes occur. A little while ago, you were a woman who had given birth to a baby. Now you are learning to be the mother of your child. Your baby, as he matures, is learning to understand and respond and know you. In addition, you and your husband, as you alternately feel discouraged and proud, tired and exhilarated, are discovering the ways in which you will grow into a family. All the turmoil and confusion and ambivalence are useful. The intensity of the experience helps to foster change and fuels the growth and development of mothers and fathers and families.

6

Adjustments in the Early Months: The Mother

Motherhood is like a new recipe—or like a new job; it takes some time to get used to it.

—ANN OAKLEY, *Becoming a Mother*

Becoming a Mother

In the early months with a baby, you may be surprised by the upheavals in your physical, mental, and emotional life. Some of these occurrences are refreshing, invigorating, and pleasurable. Others are confusing, tiring, and disturbing. Some things are happening because *you are nursing a baby;* many others happen because *you have a baby.*

Most new mothers experience fatigue and even exhaustion in the early weeks or months, regardless of the style of feeding they have chosen. If you are used to feeling energetic and getting things done, this new persistent fatigue and lack of conventional productivity can be frustrating and bewildering. Some women are amazed at the unpredictability of their days and nights, and they are disturbed by their inability to organize a reliable schedule. In addition to facing increased demands on their energy and time, many new mothers feel lonely.

Another concern for some new mothers is the public aspect of their decision to breastfeed. Nursing is a personal experience, but it is one other people notice. Although you may have thought about how you would feel nursing your baby in front of other people, the reality of breastfeeding in public may raise new issues and feelings.

Finally, your decision to breastfeed might cause you to have unexpected disagreements with persons in the medical profession. Many of the women who spoke to us described this predicament. Advice or information on breastfeeding given by medical personnel is often in conflict with what women experience, read, or hear from other nursing mothers. This surprising discovery can be confusing and disturbing.

In the early weeks, as your baby is attempting (with your help) to adjust to his new environment, you also are attempting to adjust, to carve out a style of mothering that will suit you. Breastfeeding is a part of that style. Most often a new mother's attitude toward nursing takes some time—months—to become fully formed. In the early weeks, your baby is learning and your body is adapting. It is likely that you will feel positive about some aspects of nursing, discouraged by others, and skeptical about still others. There seems to be considerable agreement among new mothers that beginning motherhood and breastfeeding are *not* what they had expected.

Making Adjustments

Fatigue

Toni Moran talked to us about some alterations she found she had to make in those early weeks.

For me, the biggest adjustment was changing gears. In the first week home, I think I was sort of stupid. I felt so great, I did everything. I was on a high. People told me I should take naps during the day. I kept thinking, "I don't want to nap. I'm not sick." Well, now I see that you can feel sicker if you don't rest. And even though I feel as though I'm taking better care of myself now, at the end of each day I still feel as though I've been run over by a truck.

There are several reasons a new mother can experience such fatigue. First, you have just completed an enormous physical task: whether you delivered vaginally or by Cesarean section, you may have undergone several hours of labor. Your body has opened up to give birth to a human being. The exact toll this takes on your body, and the time required to regain your former level of energy, is uncertain and varies from woman to woman.

In addition, you now find yourself caring for an infant who can significantly interfere with your sleep. You are constantly "on call" to meet the needs of your baby, and this can be both physically and emotionally exhausting. One mother told us that even when her newborn was napping she felt tense waiting for the cry that would indicate the baby needed her again. In those first couple of months, some mothers may have a difficult time relaxing. As the baby goes down to sleep, mom takes a look at the clock. From then until he wakes, her thinking may go something like this: *"I should take a nap, too . . . no, I should clean up the kitchen . . . no, I'll shower . . . no, then I might not hear him. What if he only sleeps twenty minutes? If he sleeps too long, will he be up all night? If I just knew how long, then maybe I could read the paper and nap."*

Certainly this mental juggling—torment?—and the tension it creates are exhausting. Several new mothers stressed the importance of getting extra sleep during the day: "Sleep when your baby sleeps. I know it bugs me that I have to nap. I'd rather spend that precious time doing something else. But without that nap I'm irritable and short with my husband, and I lose my sense of humor." Beyond the effects of feeling better, there is evidence that sleep, whether in daytime or nighttime, will increase your prolactin level. It is the hormone prolactin which is responsible for milk production. To give you a better chance of daytime sleep, some women recommend that you take the phone off the hook during nap times.

For most women, making accommodations for their new, persistent fatigue took some adjusting. "It took me a full month—and one breast infection—to realize that I should slow down, that this is a *whole new thing*. I really can't do everything I did before. I had to learn to wind down." We have been told that breast infections (localized tenderness in the breast, fever, and flulike symptoms) are most common at three months postpartum and during the Christmas season. These infections are generally associated with periods when a new mother is taking on more activities and getting less rest.

Part of winding down or changing gears can require a reordering of priorities. "The biggest thing to remember is that you have to let things go," Toni Moran told us. "I don't clean as much now. I have different priorities." In the early months, it may be difficult but necessary to realize that you rarely have the energy or the time for the endeavors you once considered "productive."

Feeling Unproductive

Joyce Steeves, who had decided to leave her full-time job after the birth of her baby, told us that during the final months of her pregnancy she had often imagined what her life at home with an infant would be like. She had expected to complete some needlepoint projects, learn how to bake bread, and finally clean out the closets.

> I even envisioned becoming very well-read. I thought I might subscribe to *Time* or *Newsweek* with some degree of confidence. I honestly thought my days at home would be rather serene and my nursing relationship with Kathryn would border on the spiritual. I can't believe how far off I was! For one thing, it takes us a long time to nurse. I may spend a total of twenty-five minutes nursing, some time for burping, some time for diaper changing, maybe some rocking-to-sleep time.

The whole process might take an hour or more. And then, in the beginning, Kathryn was ready to feed in another hour or so. If I was able to fit in a shower for myself, it was an exceptionally good day. Before I had a baby, I used to wonder what stay-at-home mothers did all day. Now I find myself wondering what *I* did all day.

The need to "accomplish something" can be strong. One mother of a two-month-old son noted the recent changes in her life: "I worked up until the birth of our baby. I was organized and productive. Suddenly there's chaos. Now I don't accomplish anything."

That intelligent and caring women need to be convinced about the practical worth of their jobs as mothers probably says something about how we value children in our society. If the careful tending of children was accepted as crucial and vital to maintaining a healthy society, mothers caring for infants would feel important and productive. The women we met who seemed to be handling this issue most successfully either already had a conviction about their roles or were redefining some terms so as to view their new responsibilities more favorably. As Lorraine Chidester, the mother of a two-month-old girl, told us, "I *am* productive. It's not productive like brain surgery is productive. It's different. My baby gains weight and thrives because I take time to hold and nurse her. Her brain is being stimulated because I talk to her and sing and smile and rock her. She might grow up secure because I take care of her. A brain surgeon? All *he* does is surgery."

Another new mother remarked that her view of herself changed during a conversation with a neighbor. The new nursing mother was complaining that she was getting nothing done, day after day. Her neighbor seemed shocked. "Getting nothing done? You're almost single-handedly keeping another human being alive! That's usually considered a big deal." It certainly helps if people around you view your mothering as a productive activity.

For some women, housework seems to become the measurement of accomplishment. "No one said, 'What a good job you're doing nursing.' The only noticeable thing I could do was housework." For women who find housework pleasurable, satisfying, and even a relaxing distraction, such activity can be valuable. For other women, who find it tedious and unpleasant, their attempts to do a good job at both house and baby can result in frustration and more fatigue. "I decided to put no demands on myself. If I did the dishes, I was to be congratulated. If everything in the house goes to hell, that's fine. This is the time of my life for baby care."

Because household responsibilities can become a source of conflict during the postpartum period, it can help if couples agree concerning their expectations. Several women felt they needed to get things straight with their husbands before they could relax about housework. Margaret Hines explained, "Before we had a baby, we both worked, we both hated cleaning, and we shared the chores. Now I've given up my job *to take care of our baby.* I did *not* give up my job to do the cleaning, shopping, cooking, laundry . . . and fit the baby care somewhere in between chores. I'm happy to get things done during the day, if there's time, but the house is not my first responsibility." A few mothers had requested that their husbands not ask, "What did you do today?" when they arrived home. "I know Tom is really just being friendly, but it's a bad question."

Decisions about Working

One of the dilemmas many women face at this time is whether to work outside the home. For some there is no debate because their families need the money. For many others, however, the issue of returning to work has much to do with the need to feel productive in a familiar and conventional way. The regularity of the hours, the sense of accomplishment, the contact with adults, and a reliable paycheck can combine to make a mother feel "normal" again. Unfortunately, it can also contribute enormously to her fatigue and to her feelings of guilt and frustration.

What's a mother to do?

After listening to a number of women describe their situations, it seems to us that flexibility is one of the most important ingredients in formulating a decision. A flexible approach helped many working

mothers to arrive at acceptable arrangements and workable routines.
Some who had arranged for a six-week or three-month leave from
their jobs felt that they needed more time once they had their babies.
They requested and were granted additional weeks or months off.
(Some companies now allow women to combine accumulated sick
leave with maternity leave, thereby providing important extra weeks
for the mother who wants more time with her infant.) Other women,
who had intended to work full-time, opted for part-time employ-
ment. One mother had taken three months of maternity leave and
then returned to work on a half-time schedule. Two months later,
however, she left her job for full-time motherhood and a one-night-
a-week teaching position.

It is important to realize that, contrary to some glowing ac-
counts in women's magazines, there are no perfect arrangements.
Whether you choose work outside the home or the daily care of your
baby, sometimes you will feel uncomfortable about your decision.
Sheila Kitzinger describes this anxiety in her book *Women as Mothers:*

> There are two contrasting mothering styles between which mothers in
> the West can choose today. On the one hand is the mother who lives
> relatively independently of the newborn baby. Having given birth to
> it, it starts its separate existence and she continues hers as before. Her
> breasts, arms and body are her own. On the other hand there is the
> other whose baby is attached to her like a limpet, who becomes herself
> the baby carrier, the baby nourisher, the baby comforter, the child's
> life growing out of hers and physically contiguous with it. There are,
> of course, many points along the continuum between these two ex-
> treme positions. Each mother may at times feel guilty or anxious that
> she is not mothering the other way. The woman who goes back to her
> job leaving the baby with other caretakers can be guilty about not
> breast-feeding and tending it herself. But so may the one who gives
> herself to the baby without restrictions. She may feel guilty about
> sudden and uncontrollable resentment at being so sucked into and
> taken over by motherhood (pp. 164–65).

It seems important to view your decision as one that may be
suitable for now but might need revision later. The choice you make,

to return to work or to care for your baby full-time, is *today's* choice. If the evidence begins to mount in favor of a change, if you discover new information about yourself or your baby or your situation, then it is appropriate for you to make new decisions.

Schedules

The mother or father who attempts to get a baby on a schedule could be facing an awesome task. In the beginning, an immature, disorganized, disoriented baby may be *incapable* of adapting to a schedule.

I was making myself crazy trying to figure out what his schedule was. I had to make myself stop writing everything down.

I get scared that I won't be able to have her on a schedule *ever*. I'll never control my life again.

The hardest thing is learning to be flexible. I'm obsessively organized and I want her to be predictable.

Yes. I've noticed a pattern now. He has a schedule . . . I just don't *like* his schedule.

Any schedule that begins to emerge may alter itself several times before settling down. It is necessary for a newborn to nurse eight to eleven times in every twenty-four-hour period. By one month, a baby may seem to be settling into a pattern of feeding every three or four hours, but at five or six weeks, he will probably begin to nurse more frequently again. If your baby seems fussier all of a sudden and anxious to nurse more frequently, don't assume your milk is drying up. He's probably going through a growth spurt. This can be disconcerting if you have just begun to believe that you've finally all settled into a schedule. At this time a baby who might have been sleeping longer stretches during the night may begin to wake

every hour and a half to two hours for feedings. That's the point of
growth spurts (see p. 86): the baby is supposed to demand more
food. By sucking at the breast more frequently, he will cause your
body to begin to produce more milk for his growing body. After a
few days of this increased sucking, your body will be making more
milk and your baby can return to less frequent nursing. (At this point
it still would not be unusual for a baby to nurse eight to eleven times
a day.) When your baby reaches three months, he'll probably experience another growth spurt. Be ready for more frequent nursings
again.

A baby's lack of schedule—both for feeding and for sleeping—
can be difficult for new parents. Understanding that his condition
makes sense biologically and developmentally may help you. It's not
a condition you should be expected to "cure." As your baby matures
and becomes capable of distraction and sustained entertainment, you
might be able to help him postpone sleeping or feeding without his
becoming miserable. But probably not yet.

Isolation

For many new mothers, there comes a time in the early weeks
when they realize that they're lonely. As one woman put it, "I taught
school until Amanda's birth. Every morning there would be thirty
second-graders around my desk with things to tell me. And I enjoyed my lunch times with other faculty members. Now it's just
Amanda and me . . . all day. I *like* her, but I miss conversation. I have
to say that taking care of her can be boring."

Women's feelings of isolation seem to result from a number of
causes. The feelings may be greater if you've been used to going out
to work and if involvement with other people filled a good part of
your day. You may feel more alone if you've just moved into a new
apartment or a new home, or if your neighborhood empties every
morning as other mothers head off to work or school. If the weather
is cold or stormy, leisurely strolls with the carriage may be impossible and your feelings of isolation may intensify. You can also find

yourself more confined and lonely if nursing outside your home is a problem for you.

Melissa Sterret, who moved into a new neighborhood shortly before her son's birth, told us she worried about several potential problems before her child's birth but never focused on loneliness:

> I wondered if I'd have enough patience for a baby, if I'd have enough stamina, if I'd love her enough. I never thought, "Will I be able to tolerate the loneliness?" One morning I got very bold and called the mother across the street to invite her in for a cup of tea. She told me she couldn't take time out because it was her upstairs day . . . she was cleaning her upstairs! For me, an upstairs day means we've probably had a tough night and I feel too tired and depressed to get dressed and go downstairs.

Although this first attempt to connect with her neighbor was not successful, Melissa suspected it was important for her to find another mother she could visit in person or on the phone. Without a doubt, the companionship of other mothers can be pleasant, rewarding, and freeing. Perhaps Virginia Barber and Merrill Maguire Skaggs are right when they suggest in *The Mother Person*, "The only segment of the community from which we can reasonably expect sustained, meaningful, sympathetic support is the one made of people in our own situation. Difficult as it may be, until we can begin to see ourselves as sharing the same basic jobs, problems and difficulties as other mothers, we have no dependable group to rely on and no community of shared feelings at all" (pp. 117–18).

Women who may have limited access to other mothers often join a lay nursing group such as La Leche League, or a postpartum discussion group, or arrange for a reunion with people from their childbirth preparation class. You might learn whether there is a baby-sitting cooperative in your neighborhood or apartment building, or you might consider organizing one. (A baby-sitting coop provides a system whereby mothers, or mothers and fathers, exchange baby-sitting responsibilities with other families.) Some mothers find that regular outings to the playground give them opportunities to meet other mothers. Even getting together one morning a week with another mother and baby can do the trick. It seems to be important to know that you have some means of escaping the isolation.

One woman, Carolyn Biles, said she had come to rely on her husband as a source of daytime adult conversation: "Mike is out of the house from 8 A.M. till almost 10 P.M. I need him to call in the middle of the day, *every* day. I honestly wasn't prepared for the isolation I'm feeling as a mother. I had read plenty that told me what to expect, but I didn't know about the isolation. And needing those phone calls from Mike . . . I feel rather insecure realizing I'm so dependent on him."

Some mothers suggested that getting out with the baby and expanding their weekday activities helped them to gain confidence. Once these women discovered they could manage with a baby in the car or on public transportation, once they felt they could nurse discreetly outside their homes, and once they got used to the idea that babies sometimes will cry in public, no matter what you do, their worlds expanded and their loneliness decreased.

Nursing in Front of Others

It is common for a new nursing mother to spend considerable time and energy trying to figure out how she can manage breastfeeding and some semblance of a social life. One woman explained that she and her husband particularly liked being with another couple who had an infant: "Most of our friends are young marrieds with no children. I don't feel I can relax and nurse in front of some of them. I sense that they are uncomfortable and I'm afraid I might embarrass them. It really is easier for me to be with someone else who has a baby." We discussed this issue with almost all the women we interviewed and discovered a wide range of reactions. From the woman who had never nursed in front of anyone except her husband, to women who felt no restrictions, we heard many self-imposed guidelines for breastfeeding in front of others:

I can nurse in front of the women in my family, but not in front of the men.

My father-in-law is like a dirty old man. If I nursed in front of him, I'd feel like I was stripping.

I'm comfortable nursing in front of our friends as long as my husband is in the room.

My unmarried girl friends seem too uncomfortable. One even told me not to nurse whenever she brought a date to our house.

I have no trouble nursing in public with strangers around. It's with certain people I know well, even my sister, that I feel uncomfortable.

One reason that mothers feel uncomfortable is the overwhelming suggestion that female breasts are predominantly and primarily sexual. Television and magazines imply that the allure of female breasts, especially if they are partially exposed, can sell cars, shaving cream, and soft drinks. This sexual aspect is underscored because we cannot match it with an equally pervasive picture of breasts as a source of nourishment and solace for a child. Before the turn of the century, men, women, and children understood that the baby's access to the mother's bared breast was natural and vital. Although female breasts were also sexually attractive, families and friends were accustomed to seeing a woman use her breasts to feed her baby. The contemporary emphasis on the sexual nature of female breasts has created the pressure to breastfeed only in privacy.

In addition to the issue of breasts as sexual objects, there is also the concern with modesty. For some women the issue of modesty persists throughout the nursing experience. Many of the mothers who spoke to us, however, suggested that time helps.

Once I felt confident about nursing—the baby seemed happy and was gaining weight; I could hold him in a nursing position without feeling awkward; I was able to hook him on very discreetly—then I started thinking about myself. I wanted to go places and be with people. If that means nursing in public places or in front of others, I can do it now. It's shocking to me how I've lost my modesty, but it does make my life easier. Someone told me I'll regain my modesty when I stop nursing.

This attitude about modesty was mentioned several times. Vivian McIntyre, a stewardess and mother of Sean, explained, "When I was a nursing mother, I wasn't very modest. I would just think, 'The baby has to eat.' And I'd feed him. Once he was weaned, I became very modest again. Now I'm sort of amazed that I could ever have been that casual about my breasts."

Some mothers begin to feel more and more relaxed, but other women, particularly in the early months, feel comfortable nursing only in private. "I'm not very open. When we visited my in-laws, I felt I should go up to the bedroom. I didn't like it, but it just seemed easiest." This dissatisfaction with isolating oneself during nursing was mentioned frequently. "It's really a pain to shut yourself away. I resent it, but I'm still too uncomfortable trying to nurse in front of other people," one mother commented. Another mother, however, pointed out the value of this isolated time with her infant: "I'm glad we can go to a quiet room and nurse. I'm more comfortable and she nurses better. It's relaxing. I don't mind. I'm not a crusader. And I believe our friends and relatives are more comfortable this way."

The reactions of your husband, your friends, or your relatives can also create some areas of conflict for you. Gwen Peterson had had a home birth, in which her husband, Larry, was very involved. When their son Brett was four weeks old, the family went out to dinner. Gwen described the incident:

We had just finished our meal in a restaurant. Our baby had been good the entire time but was beginning to fuss because it was *his* turn for dinner. I started to nurse him. We were in a booth and could hardly be seen, but my husband got annoyed with me and wanted to cancel dessert so that we could leave and I could nurse in the car. It really didn't surprise me. Larry doesn't know any nursing mothers. But I'm convinced it's just something he's got to get used to. If I go along with him, we'll never get beyond this. He's very supportive about breast-feeding, but he's ill at ease in public.

About a week later we were at another restaurant with the baby. When it was time for Brett to nurse, Larry simply asked me to change seats with him so that I wouldn't be facing the center of the room.

If a man feels uncomfortable about his wife nursing in public, he will probably convey his discomfort either explicitly or subtly. In this case, it may be useful to talk with your husband to find out what particular circumstances make him uncomfortable. Perhaps he doesn't mind your nursing in a restaurant but wouldn't want you to nurse at his company picnic. You need to explain your feelings and preferences to him. You may be able to make compromises that will ease your individual concerns. There are some new fathers who are relaxed and even grateful that nursing provides such a quick and simple solution to the hungry or fussy baby in public. Ed Simmons feels that way. His wife said, "Ed thinks of it as the original 'fast food.' The first time we had taken Carrie to a restaurant was during our vacation. I really had hoped I wouldn't have to nurse her, but either our timing was off or she was just fussy. When she started to cry, Ed said, 'Why don't you nurse her?' So I did. After that, I nursed her everywhere!''

Several women spoke about the reactions of relatives or friends that were unrelated to sexuality or modesty. Sitting down to nurse the baby in the company of others seemed to signal that it was time to discuss the issue of breastfeeding. Such remarks as the following made some new mothers feel uncomfortable or frustrated.

Are you sure you have enough milk? You just fed him an hour ago.

I don't know why you continue nursing when it's so disruptive to your sleep. If you'd start the baby on some cereal, you'd get more sleep.

You can't measure how much you're giving him. Maybe it's not enough.

My babies never cried this much. He's obviously hungry.

The poor, deprived child. She's never had a bottle.

When are you going to give her some *real* food?

Some of your friends or relatives may be critical by nature, but many of these comments are not meant to criticize your ability to care for your baby. Rather, they probably arise from a variety of concerns. It may help you to tolerate these remarks if you consider the following possibilities:

• The speaker may not understand how breastfeeding works. He or she may assume that the rules for breastfeeding are the same as those for formula feeding.

• Breastfeeding may hold certain connotations for the speaker that you don't share. For example, perhaps a grandmother remembers the switch to bottle-feeding as the modern choice, in her day, among educated, middle-class American women. She may have a difficult time understanding your desire to breastfeed.

• Remarks that focus on *you*—your need for sleep, relaxation, time off—may stem from a genuine concern for your well-being. You may find that your parents, in particular, want to protect you from any perceived difficulty.

• If your own mother or mother-in-law did not breastfeed, she may feel isolated from your experience and not know how to give you support and advice. Although she may want to pass on to you what she learned as a young mother, she may make comments that are inappropriate for your situation.

Women's reactions to such comments varied. One woman said she felt she was offending her mother by ignoring her suggestions to start cereal: "It seemed that I might be hurting her feelings by not taking her advice." Another mother remarked, "It would have been nice to have complete support, but I didn't expect it." As women gain confidence about their breastfeeding abilities, they are less disturbed by critical remarks.

Understanding the basics of breastfeeding will help you to weigh the value of advice from others and discard what does not apply. Because your confidence can be shaken at any point in your nursing experience, it's helpful to have an ally who understands and supports your commitment to breastfeeding. This ally might be your husband, a good friend, or the person answering the La Leche League hotline. What is important is that you have someplace to turn when you need to talk about any of your concerns. With accurate information and support from at least one other person, a breastfeeding mother can more easily deal with the less-than-enthusiastic opinions of others.

Part of the gain in confidence is reflected in the mother's willingness or desire to integrate nursing into her life. There are some women who conscientiously attempt to overcome their awkwardness about breastfeeding in public. When we spoke to Debbie Solomon shortly before Christmas, she was giving much thought to this issue.

> I feel as though I'll have to work on a positive attitude. We're going to a big family Christmas party. I refuse to go off by myself and nurse. I'll probably feel uncomfortable if this makes someone else uncomfortable, but I think it's worth it. I don't want to start the whole process of running and hiding. I know that I can be discreet. If it's a problem for me, if I can't get a let-down, only then will I go and sit somewhere else.

Marion Walsh, whose son was two months old, was planning an extended visit to her parents' home and had begun to consider the issue of nursing in front of them and their friends: "I'm going to start getting ready by trying to nurse in front of people in our mothers' postpartum group. I think I have to get used to this a little at a time. Maybe I won't be able to do it, but I'm going to try."

Another mother explained that she had begun shopping again

without worrying about when the baby might need to nurse: "I discovered I could easily march into a dressing room in any clothing store, nurse the baby, and then continue about my business." Another woman spoke of the first time she nursed in public: "We had gone to the zoo. I really debated about whether I could do it, but the setting—a zoo, where the focus is on nature—seemed like a safe place to try. I sat on one of the benches and nursed Christopher. A woman with a baby walked by and said, 'If my baby was ready to nurse, I'd join you.' The zoo was a good place to try it for the first time. A boy's prep school wouldn't be a good place."

If nursing in front of others makes you feel uncomfortable, here are some suggestions that may make breastfeeding in public more feasible for you.

• Choose clothing that allows you most easily to position your baby. Many women find overblouses or sweaters better than shirts that button down the front.

• One mother told us that she was concerned about how exposed she was when she lifted her shirt to place her baby to breast. Before nursing outside her home, she practiced this maneuver in front of a mirror until she was satisfied that she could manage discreetly.

• Some mothers go into another room to get their babies to start sucking. Once the baby is comfortably in place, a mother can return and finish the nursing.

• If you are uncomfortable nursing when in a group, you may choose to breastfeed your baby in another room. Often mothers feel more relaxed and less isolated if they ask someone to join them.

• In restaurants choose a seat or booth apart from or facing away from the crowds.

• Discover which stores, museums, and other public places have ladies' rooms, lounges, or other facilities with places to sit and nurse. Take advantage of these locations during your outings.

• Some women *gradually* expand the number of settings in which they will nurse. By breastfeeding in the most comfortable surroundings in the early days or weeks, and later adding new settings, a mother is able to ease herself into a wider range of comfortable nursing situations.

Women who manage to overcome the problems of first-time-in-public nursing seem to be able to go on to enjoy months of activities and travel unrestricted by their commitment to nursing. Women find they can breastfeed discreetly, even unnoticed, on buses, trains, and planes. Mothers comfortably nurse their babies in restaurants, at pools and beaches, and at the movies. Nursing may start out being the main focus of your life with a newborn. As the months go by, it becomes a part—a manageable part—of the days and nights you spend with your child.

Dealing with the Medical Profession

Within the first months of your newborn's life, you will probably be in touch with a doctor or nurse-midwife on several occasions. Barring any major complications, it is likely that your questions regarding your baby's health will deal with weight gain, sleeping, crying, and colic. The new breastfeeding mother may assume that all these areas of concern are directly related to her milk supply. It is important that the health care professional you have chosen take a broader look at the situation you present to him or her.

We think it might be valuable for you to consider the following questions when dealing with your health care practitioner:

• Did he/she study breastfeeding during medical training?

- Does he/she receive current breastfeeding information from professional journals or from literature distributed by the infant formula and baby food industry?

- Has he/she ever watched women nursing their babies?

- Is the weight gain chart he/she uses based on the norms for breastfed or bottle-fed babies?

- Does he/she routinely give advice that restricts breastfeeding and encourages the use of supplementary bottles?

The above questions are not meant to undermine your confidence in the doctor you have chosen. Instead, they are meant to help you understand the possibility that any given health care professional might *not* be an authority on infant nutrition in general and breastfeeding in particular. This does not necessarily mean you should look for another practitioner, particularly if you have confidence in the one you have chosen regarding other areas of health. It *does* mean that you need to recognize the limits of your practitioner's service.

Although I have tremendous confidence in our family practitioner regarding the health care of our children, I would not consider him the final authority in such matters as allergies or speech problems. And he would be the first to suggest that I go elsewhere for this special information. In matters of breastfeeding as well, it may be necessary for you to get your information from sources other than your pediatrician, unless he or she is up-to-date and well informed.

If you feel less than confident about the information you are receiving about breastfeeding, you can get second and third opinions elsewhere. You can gather much information from books on nursing. Other mothers who have nursed or, better still, who are presently nursing can be a terrific source of support. Attending one or more La Leche League meetings (you don't have to join to attend) can provide you with many answers and much support. Or call the

La Leche League hotline number listed in your telephone directory. There may have been a particularly helpful nurse on the maternity floor during your hospital stay. Call the hospital during her shift and talk to her. If you have a certified nurse-midwife, contact her about your breastfeeding concerns. Call your childbirth instructor. She may be able to answer your questions or lead you to some useful information.

Sometimes it can be difficult to determine whether your own pediatrician is up-to-date and supportive of breastfeeding. The claim "I'm in favor of breastfeeding" is not sufficient evidence.

One doctor who spoke to us explained his attitude toward breastfeeding:

> I definitely believe breastfeeding is the best thing *if* a woman wants to do it. Right now, though, I think some women choose it because there's such pressure out there. They feel they almost don't have a choice. If a mother comes to me with feeding problems—she's tired, the baby's nursing all the time—then I tell her to give the baby some formula and get some rest. I'm convinced that some women are looking for permission to get out of breastfeeding. I'm going to give it to them. If it's so hard on them, if they're not enjoying it, why should they continue, like martyrs?

Certainly there are some mothers who may be looking to someone in authority for permission to "get out of breastfeeding." On he other hand, there are women who may be discouraged or confused about some *aspect* of nursing and who want information and support. If, instead, their inquiries are seen as requests for permission to start formula, they are not being properly served. Here it seems important that you make yourself understood. One mother told us how she communicates with her pediatrician: "Whenever I go to her with a problem—sore nipples or constant nursings—I always start with 'Now I don't want to start him on supplementary bottles yet!' " This approach is ideal because it gives the health care professional important information about you.

If a doctor sees *breastfeeding as your problem*, he is accurate in

beginning to "cure" you of your problem by recommending formula. If, instead, he understands that you have a *particular difficulty
with breastfeeding,* the proper approach would be to give you accurate
information and support. It is your responsibility to make your
wishes clear: "I want to cut down on breastfeeding. What do I do?"
or "I want to continue breastfeeding, but I have some problems
with it."

It's possible that, even after making your intentions clear, you
might not receive accurate information. Many doctors base their
advice on feeding on information that is appropriate for formula
feeding. Several women we interviewed had chosen doctors who
were "pro-breastfeeding" but who nevertheless gave advice that was
incompatible with breastfeeding. The most common and harmful
misinformation these women received involved *restricting breastfeeding:* "You must not allow your baby to nurse any more frequently
than every three to five hours." How, then, could the mothers'
bodies make sufficient milk? What about the baby's growth spurts?
What about the fact that low-protein human milk can be digested in
an hour or so? What about the fact that nursing is useful for comforting as well as for feeding? Janet Meyers's experience demonstrates
some of the problems that can arise when a doctor bases his advice
on information about bottle-feeding.

Janet had chosen Dr. White because he was highly recommended by a friend who mentioned that he was in favor of breastfeeding and was easy to talk to. Janet went to see him for a routine
well-baby check when her son was two weeks old. At that time he
told her that feedings should be spaced at three- to five-hour intervals. In the following two weeks, this advice seemed to present no
difficulty for Janet's son. He was content to nurse every three or four
hours. Gradually, however, a problem seemed to be developing.
The baby was becoming cranky, crying frequently, and waking often
during the night. When he was five weeks old, Janet and her husband became concerned. Janet suggested that perhaps she should
nurse the baby more often. Her husband insisted that they stick to
the schedule Dr. White had set. "We're paying him good money.
We're not going to ignore his advice."

Because Janet was worried, she took her son back to see Dr. White. During this visit, the doctor determined that the five-week-old baby was suffering from colic, and he prescribed medication. The medication contained bentyl (to relieve muscle spasms in the intestines and stomach) and phenobarbital (to act as a sedative). In the following week, Janet gave her son the medication when he could not be consoled. He would eventually calm down and usually fall asleep.

At the end of this week, Janet, her husband, and her son spent Saturday with friends who also had a nursing newborn. During this twelve-hour period Janet began to question her own breastfeeding style. She observed that her friend nursed her infant much more frequently than she did and, occasionally, seemed to nurse the baby simply to quiet him.

When we talked to Janet on that Monday, she already had begun to experiment with the information she had received from her friend. During the day on Sunday, Janet had nursed her baby whenever he seemed to indicate an interest. Not surprisingly, she claimed that Sunday was the first day that he didn't seem to suffer from colic.

While visiting her friend, Janet learned two things that had encouraged her to try frequent nursings. First, she had been told that human milk is digested much more easily and quickly than formula. Thus her son could actually be hungry in less than three hours. Second, she had been told that every once in a while a baby goes through a growth spurt and requires more food. Thus, though he *had* been content with three-hour feedings, by the time he reached five weeks of age, he was requiring more and demanding more. This behavior had been diagnosed as colic. The pediatrician's recommended schedule actually interfered with the breastfeeding because the mother's body will produce a greater milk supply only as the result of the baby's increased nursing.

Most women today will find themselves, at some point, turning to their obstetricians, nurse-midwives, pediatricians, and/or family practice doctors for information related to breastfeeding. Since an enormous number of these professionals received little or no training in breastfeeding issues, have never breastfed a baby, and do not even have one of the current texts on breastfeeding in their offices, it could be difficult or impossible to get up-to-date, practical information from them. Fortunately, there are a number of health care professionals who are doing something about this.

We learned of one pediatrician who arranged to have someone join his practice for the purpose of providing breastfeeding information and answering questions about nursing. The young woman, Susan Campbell, is an R.N. and has nursed her own child. She maintains a library and a file on breastfeeding issues and keeps informed through current, related journals. On Monday evenings she holds a class on breastfeeding for couples who are close to their due dates. Grandparents are also invited to attend this class. Working closely with the pediatrician, Susan calls a woman the day after she gives birth. If it's been a hospital birth, Susan will call again the day the woman arrives at home. A program is suggested to the new mother that will help her avoid such problems as sore nipples and engorgement. The pediatrician sees the newborn at one week of age.

Susan is available to make home visits or meet the mother and baby at the doctor's office. She is also available to answer questions by phone every afternoon. She handles no medical problems. Nor, says Susan, is it her job to tell a woman what to do. Instead, she provides information about infant development, the nature of breastmilk, and how breastfeeding works. The pediatrician refers all questions related to nursing to Susan, who believes that "with accurate information and understanding, a woman can decide what's best."

In the end, you're the mom. None of the professionals, nor any other mother, will know your baby as you do. It's important for you to pay close attention to that baby, apply the information you receive, and make thoughtful decisions. A baby who, at three months of age, becomes cranky and cries more frequently could be going through a growth spurt and need more nursing, or he could be suffering from an earache. At such times, you need a good pediatrician or family practitioner *and* accurate information about breastfeeding. It's not so terrible if you can't get both in the same place.

7

Adjustments in the Early Months: Siblings

*And why would a mother
want a new baby, unless the
old one were not good enough?*

SARA BONNETT STEIN, *The
New Baby*

WHEN a family of three becomes a family of four, life becomes more complicated for each family member. Suddenly, mother and father each have two children to respond to. The older child not only has to develop a relationship with a new brother or sister, but he is also affected by that sibling's relationship with each of his parents. For some children the experience of having and becoming a sibling is likely to be among the most stressful of early childhood. With the arrival of a new baby, familiar routines and relationships take on unexpected dimensions. Mommy's lap and daddy's attention may not be as available after the new baby's birth, even though they are more needed than ever.

Mother nursing the new sibling is but one of a host of changes the toddler or preschooler must adapt to. Those changes began even before the new baby arrived. During pregnancy, mother's familiar body changed, and so did her moods and energy level. And that was just the beginning. For your older child, a new brother or sister is also likely to cause rearrangements in existing family relationships and in familiar routines. Some changes in routine that often occur for the young child around the time that a new baby is born include:

- A separation from the mother for childbirth
- Father's being unusually busy with new responsibilities
- A move to a bigger house or apartment
- Giving up a familiar crib
- Getting a new bed
- Changing bedrooms
- Sharing a bedroom
- Being toilet-trained
- Giving up nursing, a bottle, or pacifier
- Starting nursery school

How well each child manages these changes partially depends on his age when the baby is born.

It's easy to assume that any troublesome changes you observe in your older child are directly related to your having and nursing a new baby. The three-and-a-half-year-old who begins to stutter and stammer or the four-year-old who displays emotional outbursts and becomes loud and rambunctious may appear to be reacting to the changed situation. In fact, these behaviors are typical of children at these ages, regardless of whether there is a new baby in the house.

Nonetheless, children usually do show reactions to the arrival of a sibling. These may include remarks of disapproval about the baby, aggression toward the baby, or less direct behaviors such as sleep problems, attention-seeking, and bed-wetting.

One young mother recalled that when her baby, Erica, was seven weeks old, her older daughter, Diane, remarked, "How long is Erica going to stay with us?" Then she added, "I kind of wish we had gotten a dog instead."

This mother commented that Diane's first job was to adjust to a new baby who took up a lot of time and wasn't much fun. Then, just as she got used to the presence of this demanding new resident, the baby became a charming three-month-old. Erica laughed and cooed and got a lot of attention from neighbors, parents, and grandparents. Although she was also more fun for Diane, her popularity posed a new challenge. Diane started wetting her bed about that time.

No matter how hard you try to understand and sympathize with the difficulties your older child is having adjusting to the baby, you will not be able to make the difficulties disappear. Furthermore, you will sometimes—or often—feel furious at your older child for having those difficulties. Mothering two or more children is very hard work. It is hard physical work and hard emotional work. You are on the go from the time your first child awakens in the morning until your last child goes to sleep at night. And you are on call twenty-four hours a day. You are bound to be tired and impatient at times, regardless of your best intentions.

One mother, Colleen Stewart, told us,

> When the baby cried and I was trying everything to calm him, I didn't want Jennie asking me over and over if I'd color with her. When I would try to hurry to get Jennie out of the bath before the baby woke up, I got furious at her for moving slowly. It was as if I couldn't stand her being a kid. I felt strained to my limits caring for the baby. I would hear myself cooing at the baby as I changed his diapers, then snapping at Jennie to hurry and get dressed. I heard myself and I didn't like it.

This mother's feelings are not so different from those we heard from others. Mothers reported an array of intense, unexpected feelings provoked by the older—formerly dearest—children. Much of the intensity seems to diminish when baby care takes less time, when mother gets more sleep, and when everyone adjusts to the new routines with a baby in the house. Colleen said four things helped her work through and moderate her feelings. First was the passage of time—things got easier as the baby reached eight to ten weeks of age. Second, she talked to friends and learned that they too had experienced, and their families had survived, the same intense feelings. Third, she was able to talk with her husband, who acted as Jennie's advocate and helped Colleen regain her perspective that Jennie was still a young child who had needs that had to be met, too. Finally, a friend suggested that Colleen set aside fifteen or twenty minutes a day when they would do together some activity that Jennie chose.

Colleen concluded, "The effect of setting aside some time was good for both of us. Jennie would start planning early in the day what we would do during our special time, and I would feel totally free to play when I knew it was for a limited time. Otherwise I felt tense about playing dolls when the dishwasher had to be emptied or sitting down to color when I had phone calls that had to be made. It was not the only time we spent together, but it was our escape valve."

When the Baby Nurses

Curiosity

The mothers we interviewed had older children who were from eighteen months to seven years old when the new baby was born. The majority of the older siblings, however, were between about two and four. Several mothers described their children as curious about nursing at first; later, they took it in stride as part of life with baby. The children's initial curiosity seemed to be related to their mothers' breasts, their own breasts, and the mechanics of nursing. They wanted to know how the milk got into the breast, how the milk came out, and why some people had milk in their breasts and others didn't. For example, some children were curious about the fact that their dads and grandmothers didn't have milk for the baby.

One mother told us her two-and-a-half-year-old son Kevin

stared at her once as she was putting on her bra. She told him, "This is where Judy eats." A few weeks later, when Kevin saw his grandmother putting on her bathing suit, he pointed to her breasts and asked, "What's that?" "Part of my body," the grandmother replied. "For Judy to eat?" Kevin queried.

Each child tries to understand what nursing is all about by watching, asking questions, and attempting to integrate this new experience into his experiences of the world. One seven-year-old named Tina, who had never seen anyone breastfeed, giggled and seemed embarrassed the first time she saw her mother, Anne, nurse her newborn brother. Although her mother had told her before the baby's birth that she would be giving him breastmilk, Tina had thought breastmilk was given in a bottle. She hadn't realized it meant an entirely different way of feeding.

When Anne understood Tina's confusion, they talked about breastfeeding and what breasts were for. Tina asked, "Did you do that with me?" Anne said, "No." Then they talked about all the other ways mothers and babies can be close. By the time the baby was ten days old, Tina seemed to understand and be at ease with her mother's nursing. She would sit nearby and continue whatever she had been doing without paying much attention.

Other Reactions

When we asked what children usually did while mothers nursed the baby, mothers mentioned a variety of behaviors. They described children as

- Wanting to be close to mother and baby
- Wanting the mother to read, sing, or put a puzzle together with them
- Wanting the mother to get them something to eat or a Band-Aid for a real or imagined scratch
- Pretending to nurse or bottle-feed a doll or stuffed animal
- Getting into mischief

- Ignoring the nursing
- Asking to nurse

Regardless of what the child was doing during nursing, there was usually a lot of activity. Mothers rarely seem to have the opportunity to nurse their second babies in the calm, quiet, peaceful way they remembered having had with their first. One mother wondered aloud what the experience of nursing was like for the younger baby: "When my first baby nursed, everything was so quiet. I'd sit on the couch and barely a word would pass my lips. With my second, everything is different. I sit down to nurse and have to jump up to get something for my older daughter. I sit down again and have to shout at her to get down from the cupboards. I always wonder how the baby feels being nursed by a perpetual motion/shouting machine."

Even when the older child is calm and not mischievous during nursing times, mothers reported they still had to stay tuned into the sibling's activities. Gone were the days of lying down in the middle of the afternoon to nurse the baby and falling asleep together. Many mothers found that they now really enjoyed the nighttime feedings when the house was peaceful.

Aside from mischievousness, mothers found that their toddlers and preschoolers interrupted nursings by their desire to be in the same chair or even in the mother's lap. One sixteen-month-old liked to hold her mother's breast up while the baby nursed. Despite such good intentions, the little ones can't help but wiggle, get up and down, and crowd into the smallest space. And despite the mothers' best intentions, they sometimes (or often) can't help getting tense, annoyed, or downright angry.

Jane Ungerleider, mother of two, a four-year-old boy and a ten-month-old girl, said,

> I used to read to Jimmy or talk to him while I was nursing Laurie. But once she got to four months, she got so distractible I couldn't even talk. Sometimes Jimmy insists on trying to get her attention while she's nursing. I get annoyed and say, "Go in your room and play. I'll be

done in a few minutes!" If he's in a funny mood, that doesn't work, and he continues his antics. Sometimes I get furious and yell at him.

Of course, I always feel lousy when I do that because I realize he probably is too young to understand or care. What works best is if I remember to give him a warning before I start nursing. He usually behaves pretty well if I say, "Jimmy, the baby's tired. I'm going to nurse her and put her down for a nap. Then I can play with you."

Several mothers described delightful nursing routines that included mother, baby, and older child. One mother said that whenever she nursed three-month-old Sylvia, nineteen-month-old Anya would bottle-feed her baby doll, put powder and cut-down Pampers on her, then put her to sleep at the end of Sylvia's bassinet. Anya used so many Pampers for her doll that her aunt gave her a box of them for her birthday.

You may find that you can nurse with few interruptions during most of the day. Many mothers explained that it was the late afternoon or early evening nursings that presented a problem. The baby may have difficulty settling down to nurse, the older child is likely to be tired and demanding, and you may wish you were at the end of your day, but you are still facing dinner and bedtime routines. Whenever you find that the presence or demands of your older child are making nursing more difficult, you might try some of the following measures:

• Tell your older child that you will soon begin nursing the baby. Ask him if he needs anything before you start. Many young children do much better if they are forewarned about a change in activity.

• Get a snack ready for each of you before you sit down to nurse. You may both benefit from something to eat and drink.

• If your older child enjoys a favorite television show each afternoon, arrange to join him for that occasion and nurse your baby then.

• You might choose to sit on the couch or your bed when you nurse. That way your older child has the freedom and space to sit close to you. Although he may come and go several times during a nursing, there will not be the issue of whether there is room for him.

• Before you settle in for this nursing, you can set up something nearby for your older child to do. Whether it's coloring, a puzzle, stickers, blocks, or doll play, having an activity at hand can reduce the chances that you will need to interrupt this feeding.

When Your Older Child Asks to Nurse

Most of the pregnant mothers we met dreaded the possibility that their older child might want to nurse again. Most did not wish to resume nursing an already weaned toddler or preschooler, yet they felt nervous about refusing such a bid for closeness.

Although we met one or two other mothers who were willing to nurse an older child, most hoped to discourage their child's interest without being hard on him. As one mother reported,

> Initially Molly, who was two, was always on my lap when I nursed Pam. She'd announce, "I want to eat Mommy's breast, too." She tried to nurse about three times, but she seemed to have forgotten how to suck. I thought if she got some milk she'd realize she didn't like it. I didn't want her to start nursing again. So I squirted some milk into her mouth. She sort of screwed up her face. She didn't like it. Now she says, "It's yukky!" When I nurse Pam, Molly says, "I have to feed my baby now," and she gives her doll a bottle.

We heard variations of this story again and again. Once given permission to try nursing, many children become embarrassed when they are held to the breast and decide they don't want to try. Some do try but can't remember how to suck. And others suck but do not like the taste of the breastmilk. In most instances, one try is enough to satisfy the child's urge.

Sometimes, this pattern does not hold. Some children do like the milk or sensations of nursing. Some like being a baby again. Some will continue to ask to nurse once they have been permitted to try. This is when the mother's resourcefulness is put to the test. But rest assured that you do not have to start nursing again to maintain your child's love. You can be honest with him and say something like "You're three years old now, and I feel funny when you suck on my breast like a baby. You can try once to see what it's like, but you're too big to be nursed."

You probably feel the same about your toddler or preschooler nursing as you would about his using a bottle again. Once children have moved on developmentally, the thought of their regressing is not appealing. Being honest about your feelings with your child is preferable to making up stories or excuses such as "There won't be enough milk for the baby." It is important, however, to consider why your child wants to try nursing again.

- Is he just curious about the process? If so, you can show him how the milk spurts out of the many holes in your nipple. You can let him taste some from a cup. You can point out how the baby's whole face is used in sucking. You can share your amazement about how well breastfeeding works to feed babies.

- Does your child want to nurse to be as close to you as the baby? If so, you can invite him to sit with you while you nurse. You can have him choose a story to read together while nursing. You can find times to share with him alone while the baby is occupied.

- Does your child want to be the baby? If so, you can find other ways to "baby" him. You can rock him, sing to him, or snuggle in bed. You can assure him that he is both your big boy and your baby—that even grown-ups like to be babies sometimes. Everyone likes to be held and taken care of. You can encourage him always to tell you when he needs you because you want to take care of him. You can also emphasize how glad you are that he is four now so he can share experiences that babies are too young to enjoy.

• Does your child want to nurse because sucking is so much fun? Try lollipops, popsicles, pieces of ice, or straws for drinking milk or juice. You can get him one of these oral treats before you start nursing the baby.

• Is he bored while you nurse? Think of an activity you can do together or he can do near you while you are nursing the baby. Tell him beforehand that it is time for the baby to eat so you'll be busy for a short time; then you can do something together.

The basic principles of weaning described in Chapter 10 may also be useful in dissuading your older child from repeatedly asking to nurse. In particular, find substitutes for nursing that are good from your child's point of view. When possible, arrange your nursing routine to satisfy your older child's needs for attention, closeness, warmth, and accessibility, whether or not you nurse him.

As in weaning, if you are certain in your own mind that you do not want to nurse your older child, you will find your denials can be firm without being harsh or rejecting. After a short transition period of extra persistence and attention on your part, life should settle into a routine and your older child will understand that mommy's love and attention are still his even though mommy's breasts are for baby.

Nursing the Second Time Around

When we asked mothers how nursing the second baby was different from nursing the first, most women described differences in the babies and their styles of nursing and also in their own feelings and attitudes toward nursing.

Sharon Thomas, a mother of two boys, aged eighteen months and six years, said,

My first experience with nursing was a disaster. It was a series of misunderstandings. Someone had sold me on a four-hour schedule, and I thought the baby would be immorally spoiled if I fed it more often. I nursed two weeks and stopped. In the four and a half years between babies, my pediatrician and I both learned a lot. My second baby seemed to nurse continually the first month—while he was awake and while he slept. When I'd take a nap in the afternoon, I'd attach him and we'd both doze off. I had a special situation; it was summer and we had two weeks at the beach with a mother's helper, so I had no responsibilities. Besides, I knew by then how short a time a baby is content to just lie in your arms. So to just sit and nurse for a month was heaven.

Another mother of two girls, aged three months and nineteen months, said,

I'm so much more relaxed this time. With my first baby I felt very funny about breastfeeding. I always thought I'd feel like a cow. The only reason I did it the first time was my midwife said I really should for a week. This time I've been more relaxed. I knew what to expect. I also got a good breast pump (a Loyd-B) for going out in the evening and for when we're having people for dinner. Carla, my baby, doesn't mind the bottle.

A mother with a daughter, twenty-seven months, and a son, five months, said,

Brian is a fussy nurser. He started getting distracted by the time he was one or two weeks old. I can't even read while I nurse. He lets go of my nipple all the time. Shelley was different. Once she was attached, she'd stay on no matter what. Shelley always nursed herself to sleep. When she was an infant we never had the experience of tucking her in, kissing her goodnight, and leaving. She'd scream for an hour and never settle herself without comforting. With Brian, we can put him in his crib and leave. He fusses a minute, finds his thumb, and goes to sleep.

Another commented, "My first son was a good nurser from the beginning. He never had any problems. But my second son had a hard time, especially the first week. He seemed to have trouble finding the nipple. It took us several weeks to get things working smoothly."

One mother told us that nursing her third baby was the hardest because her two older children were always on the go and needed her to chaperone and chauffeur them. So she and the baby went to soccer games, swim meets, and Brownie investitures. Because the baby was often content to sleep in her Snugli, the mother frequently skipped nursings and ended up with two breast infections.

Mothers commonly mentioned the following differences in their own physical experiences of nursing a first and later time:

- Many mothers experienced stronger "after birth" cramps the second time.
- Nipples were noticeably sorer the first time for some mothers and the second time for others.
- The initial pain when the baby latches on seemed stronger the second time for a number of mothers.
- Milk seemed to come in more quickly the second time for many mothers.
- Some mothers reported feeling the let-down response both more quickly and more strongly their second time.
- Many mothers felt less engorged the second time.
- Most mothers reported less leaking the second time.
- One mother with flat nipples had to pinch and roll them for one month to get them to stand erect with her first baby but not at all with the second.

Tandem Nursing

Nursing siblings who are not twins, often called tandem nursing, is no longer an unheard-of phenomenon. Some mothers stumble into tandem nursing when an older child is not yet weaned before the baby's birth or when the older child who had been weaned resumes nursing after the newborn's arrival. Other mothers intentionally decide to continue the nursing relationship with the older child because he seems too young to be deprived of the closeness and security nursing provides.

Deborah Jones is a mother who did not wean her son before her daughter's birth. "Mark was about fourteen months old when I was surprised to discover that I was six weeks pregnant," Deborah began. When she asked her obstetrician if continuing to nurse Mark would be a problem, he said no. "I was glad," Deborah told us. "Mark wasn't ready to be weaned. He was still nursing four or five times a day. I'd never even left him with a bottle. I really didn't want to wean him under pressure. I just assumed it would happen gradually in the next few months." Deborah explained that she never envisioned herself nursing two babies.

Yet the first and second trimesters came and went and Mark was still nursing. Deborah's thoughts about weaning were suddenly interrupted when she was seven months pregnant. She and her family flew to Boston to be with her dying father. "After we returned home, I realized there was never going to be a good time to wean. By then it was just a month until the baby was due. I didn't feel it was fair to Mark to stop nursing then. That was when I realized," Deborah explained, "that I would be tandem nursing."

The first day Deborah was home after her daughter Amy's birth, Mark wanted to nurse when he saw the baby nurse. His father distracted him by reading him a story. Then Deborah nursed him when Amy was finished.

I began experiencing an internal struggle that continued as long as I nursed both children. I worried about having enough milk for Amy. Even though I knew intellectually that I had enough milk, I was anxious about it. I was most relaxed the times Amy nursed well and went to sleep before Mark asked to nurse.

After a few weeks, Mark's nursing tapered down to one or two times a day. Some days he missed altogether, but usually he liked to nurse when he woke up in the morning.

When I asked Deborah to describe how Mark had moved from one nursing a day to being totally weaned, she said it was hard to remember because the transition had been so gradual. For several months she had followed the recommendation of the La Leche League—she never offered him her breast, but she never refused either. Sometimes she did postpone his requests by saying, "This is not a good nursing time, this is breakfast time." Suddenly he stopped asking. Sometime between the ages of twenty-seven and twenty-eight months, Mark weaned himself, about five months after the baby's birth.

If you are considering tandem nursing, you will want to know:

• If you become pregnant, there is usually no need to wean your nursing child hastily.

• You will produce colostrum toward the end of your pregnancy and in the immediate postpartum period.

• You can nurse both children without impairing the nourishment of your new infant. Although you should usually give your new baby the first opportunity at your breast, varying the order somewhat will assure that he also gets those nutrients that are more prevalent in the milk which comes at the end of a feeding.

• You must take care of yourself by eating properly, drinking plenty of fluids, and getting enough rest and support to manage the added demands tandem nursing will entail.

✥ 8 ✥

Working and Nursing

*I don't know which I'm more
proud of at the end of the
day—my work or my two
little bottles of milk.*

—A WORKING MOTHER

YOU DON'T have to stop breastfeeding if you return to work—even if you work full-time. As we talked with women about their experiences, we were amazed by the variety of working-nursing patterns individuals had developed. Some women work full-time and express breastmilk during the day to be given to their babies while they are gone. Others work full-time but do not express milk. Their babies are given formula while the mothers are away and nursed when the mothers are home. Many women choose to work part-time, some expressing milk, others not.

If you begin to work while continuing to nurse, your experience will be much like that of a mother who is just beginning to breastfeed. You must develop new nursing routines and be aware of your own and your baby's responses to the changes. Developing a smooth pattern that is mutually satisfying may take time and perseverance.

One of your first concerns may be the best time to return to your job. There really are no hard and fast rules. Some women can go back as soon as two weeks after birth and continue to nurse, but this situation is rare. At two weeks your milk supply is still getting established. That means that slight variations in your schedule will greatly affect the amount of milk you produce. After eight to twelve weeks of nursing on demand, however, your supply will be more stable and will not immediately drop if you miss a feeding. This will give you more freedom to maintain your supply while separated from your baby whether or not you plan to pump.

Most women need a couple of months to rest and feel good physically, to relax and get to know their new babies, and to establish comfortable nursing. An advantage to waiting a full six months before returning to work is that by then your baby will probably be eating some solids and beginning to drink from a cup. Thus you can continue nursing without having to fulfill all your baby's nutritional needs.

Perhaps the best advice for the pregnant woman planning maternity leave is to try to arrange a flexible timetable. You really will not know how you will feel about returning to work until after your baby is born. Aside from the physical issues of recovering from giving birth and building up a good nursing relationship, many women are surprised to find that they do not feel emotionally ready to leave their babies as soon as they had expected.

One mother remembered standing at the bus stop her first morning back to work wondering, "Why am I doing this?" She said that repeatedly during her first weeks back at work she would find herself thinking about her baby. Suddenly her milk would flow. "Missing her made the dull days at the office harder to take. Even good days I'd race home to see her." In retrospect, she continues, "I could have stayed out longer than two months. When I got back, nothing had changed."

The conflict most women feel when the time comes to leave their babies is captured in Tina Horwitz's account of her first day back at school. She had taught for twelve years before Adam's birth, and she really enjoyed teaching. When Adam was four months old, she reported for her first day at a new school. Her husband, Bill, was going to take Adam to the baby-sitter's house.

That first day of school Tina walked into the building with tears in her eyes. She couldn't concentrate on a word during the teachers' orientation conference that morning. She remembers feeling sad and lonely when she went to the classroom to prepare for the children's arrival the next day. A note on the blackboard caught her eye. Bill had scribbled, "Adam is fine. I spent an hour with him at the baby-sitter's and he was laughing when I left." Tina began to relax.

For some women the question is not so much when to return to their jobs as how to restructure their jobs to complement their lives as nursing mothers. One way to do this is to work fewer days. For example, one woman who worked at a pharmacy returned to work three days a week when her son Jeffrey was three months old. She found a baby-sitter a few blocks from her job so she could nurse him just before work, at lunchtime, and again after work. This worked well because Jeffrey had already put himself on a four-hour schedule. Many babies do not do this by two months, and indeed, many never do.

Another way to restructure work is to do some at home. Beth Morrison, who is a graphic designer, began working at home when her son Kyle was two months old. She had her drawing board all set up, and she sat down to work the instant he fell asleep for naps and in the evenings. When she had a lot to do, she nursed Kyle and then took him to his grandmother's. This gave Beth extra blocks of time. Once a week Beth took her work to the office.

"Being at home worked well for us," Beth reported, "because Kyle nursed so frequently—every hour and a half in the beginning. When I was pregnant I had heard that breastfed babies like to feed more often, but I thought that meant every three hours instead of every four. Instead, he'd nurse for fifteen to twenty minutes every hour or hour and a half." When Kyle was six months old Beth began to go to the office three days a week. She started weaning him then by just nursing him mornings and nights and giving him formula in between. When we spoke to Beth, Kyle was eight months old and Beth was planning to start working five days a week, although she was not sure she would continue. She had discovered that she loved working part-time. "I live a schizophrenic existence between work and home," Beth exclaimed. "When I'm home I'm totally so—I can't imagine anything else. When I'm at work—I'm totally there.

I love my two worlds. I'll try working full-time, but I'm not sure I'll last."

The working-nursing arrangement that surprised us the most, however—because we hadn't realized it could be possible—was one described by two mothers who each worked three full days a week, Tuesday, Wednesday, and Thursday, and stayed home four days, Friday through Monday. Neither of these women expressed milk while at work. Both babies were given formula by their baby-sitters about three times a day for each of the three days that their mothers were away. Yet the mothers nursed their babies mornings, evenings, and nights on work days and exclusively breastfed their babies the days they were home.

One of those mothers said her baby had to nurse frequently on Fridays to build up her supply. By the end of the weekend, her milk supply was usually up and the baby nursed less frequently, yet on Tuesdays, when she returned to work, she did not pump, leak, or feel excessively full. The other mother, however, did feel full on Tuesdays and had to change her breast pads frequently. But she never felt unduly uncomfortable. Although many mothers would not choose this schedule, it fit the needs of these two. It is interesting to realize how adaptive our bodies can be.

Sometimes strict job requirements eliminate your voice in the decision regarding how many hours a week you will work or whether you can complete some work at home. In a surprising number of instances, however, more flexibility exists than is immediately apparent. In the course of writing this book, we met women who have chosen to be part-time nurses, secretaries, cashiers, saleswomen, accountants, psychologists, graphic designers, librarians, family practice residents, writers, childbirth educators, and lawyers. They have worked from two to thirty-two hours a week. Many have planned to increase their hours as their children get older.

Arranging for flexibility in work schedule and workplace can be a great advantage for nursing because mothers miss fewer feedings. Thus their supply of milk is more likely to remain adequate. Whether the mother works part of each day or three full days, her time with the baby—and with the baby sucking—will build up the volume lost when nursings are missed. Even if the mother pumps while she is gone, her supply may diminish because the pump is never as efficient as the baby. Remember, milk is produced by the law of supply and demand. The more sucking stimulation, the more milk there will be.

Even when their jobs or financial considerations do not allow for part-time or flexible scheduling, many women continue to breast-feed after they return to full-time work away from home. Both your body and your baby can adapt to a routine based on part-time nurs-ing. If you nurse on a regular schedule, even though it is not around-the-clock, your body will respond by producing milk on that regular basis. Thus, many working women choose to breastfeed their babies only in the evening, during the night, and in the early morning. Many neither nurse nor pump during the day at work. Provided that a good milk supply has already been established, this part-time nurs-ing routine can continue indefinitely.

One mother, Lisa Jordan, returned to work full-time when her daughter Shannon was three months old. She told us that she nursed mornings and evenings. This routine worked well until at seven months Shannon weaned herself from the morning nursing. "As long as Shannon nursed twice a day, my supply stayed up," ex-plained Lisa. "But when she got down to once a day, I no longer produced enough milk to satisfy her in the evening." Other mothers are able to continue to nurse just once a day. The point is that despite the body's great flexibility, there are some limits to its adaptability. Some factors that seem to affect how well nursing goes once mothers return to work are the baby's age when mother returns to work, the baby's temperament, the mother's desire to continue, how much time she has for nursing, and, when expressing milk, the regularity of her expressing.

A crucial variable, of course, is the amount of support you receive from your husband, baby-sitter, co-workers, and friends. The more people you have behind you, the more manageable your task should be. Your child's sitter, surprisingly, can have a big influ-ence on how well nursing and working go together. You would like someone who is sympathetic to breastfeeding, understands or is willing to learn something about it, and will follow your directions about issues like trying not to feed your baby just before you return, if you prefer nursing him then. When nursing and working, some extra considerations may influence your search for ideal baby-sitting arrangements.

• Discuss nursing with your prospective sitter. Find out if she has taken care of other breastfed babies. Several mothers reported that their sitters were very helpful. One mother, for example, was bringing the sitter eight-ounce bottles of expressed milk for her four-month-old son. But he was not drinking that much at a feeding. So the sitter advised her to divide it into two bottles, then into three, so they would not waste any. Other sitters have been willing to take time to help a young breastfed baby adjust to a bottle or to work with an older infant on using a cup.

• You may want someone who can bring your baby to you at work to be nursed. One pediatrician involved in research took her baby and baby-sitter to work with her. She found a college student to be both baby-sitter and research assistant. While the baby slept in a port-a-crib in her mother's office, the college student did filing and some clerical work. When the baby woke up, the mother nursed her, then the college student took her for a walk or played with her. This arrangement continued through the first year, although the college student had less and less "research" time as the baby grew older.

• You may want to find a sitter near where you work so you can nurse your baby at lunchtime or during breaks. Many countries of the world—not including the United States—have enacted International Labor Organization (part of the United Nations) guidelines guaranteeing nursing breaks to working nursing mothers. Perhaps as increasing numbers of working women continue to nurse their babies, we can lobby for this legislation here.

If you do intend to continue to breastfeed once you have returned to work, you need to consider

- Whether you wish to nurse your baby when you're home and leave formula when you are gone.
- Whether you wish to leave breastmilk for your baby while you are away. If so, you will need to express, or pump, your milk.

Leaving Formula While You Are Away

If you will be away from your baby when he must eat, you must decide whether or not you want to provide breastmilk. This is a personal decision, based partially on your own and your husband's feelings about breastmilk, formula, and nursing, your baby's age, your baby's tolerance of formula, your family's history of allergies, and whether your job allows you the freedom to pump.

If you plan to leave formula for your baby while you are gone, you will want to wean your baby from some feedings and substitute bottles of formula. This will help your body adapt to the demand for less milk while you are gone. Although it can be accomplished in less time, allowing four to seven days to make each substitution will give your body and your baby the time to make a gradual transition.

One month before returning to work, Diane Nelson began to wean Luke, who was then two months old, from the daytime feedings. The first week she dropped their noon nursings, the next week the 4 P.M. ones, and finally the 9 A.M. ones. Each time she dropped a nursing her breasts took a couple of days to adjust. The first day they felt very full at the time she typically would have nursed, but within about three days her body seemed to have stopped producing milk at that time.

Diane described how difficult the transition to the bottle had been at first. "Luke refused it. He screamed. I was really emotional." Diane called Luke's pediatrician, who suggested expressing some milk into a bottle before starting the feeding. He suggested that Diane begin a feeding by breastfeeding Luke, then after a few minutes switching to the breastmilk in a bottle. After a couple of days,

Diane switched to formula in a bottle, and within a week Luke was taking that without complaint.

Another recommendation for the common challenge of helping your baby adjust to the bottle is offered by lactation consultant JoAnne Scott:

> Do not think that *you* must offer bottles to get the baby used to them. If you already have offered bottles, and your baby has had no trouble adjusting, wonderful. But many mothers have found their babies adamantly refuse to accept bottles from them. The key phrase here is "from them." Many breastfed babies will accept a bottle from someone else much more readily than they will from their mother and, if you think you must get your baby "ready" for the babysitter, you may cause yourself unnecessary anxiety.
>
> If you have chosen a babysitter who is familiar with breastfed babies, she will know this, and be prepared to spend extra time with the baby the first days getting the baby used to the bottle. Most babies quickly adapt to the idea that "this woman feeds me this way, but mother feeds me that way." Long after the baby has happily adjusted to the bottle from the sitter he may continue to refuse one from you. Consider that to be a positive sign: the baby has a very clear idea which one of you is his mother. (Personal communication)

The following tips can help you maintain your milk supply if you choose to work and not pump while you are gone:

• Nurse your baby exclusively for three months, if possible, to assure the stability of your milk supply.

• Give your body four to seven days to adjust to the elimination of a particular feeding.

• While at work, hand express some milk a few minutes each day to stimulate your breasts even if you are not saving the expressed milk for your baby.

• Nurse frequently while you are home.

- Consider taking your baby to bed at night to increase your contact and sucking stimulation.

- Eat well, get plenty of rest, and drink a lot of fluids.

- Watch your breasts to identify any plugged ducts. These hardened, pealike lumps can be caused by insufficiently emptying the milk ducts. This may happen if you are not nursing for long periods of time or if your nursing schedule is erratic. Plugged ducts can lead to breast infections if ignored. If you find a local area of tenderness and a small lump within either breast, use moist heat and massage to try to move the blockage down the duct. Have the baby nurse frequently and first from the affected breast. Position the baby with his chin near the tender spot as this exerts maximal pressure on the blockage. Continue these measures until the duct flows freely. This may take a few days. Get extra rest and eat well during this period.

Leaving Breastmilk While You Are Away

If you want to leave breastmilk for your baby while you are at work, you will need to collect your milk by expressing it by hand or using a breast pump. If you plan to try pumping, it is a good idea to begin practicing before you return to work. At first, you will feel clumsy, regardless of the method you use, but with practice you will become proficient. You will find more information on pumps, pumping, and fostering a let-down in Chapters 2 and 4. You will probably be disappointed by the tiny amount you get the first times you pump. Many women only get one-quarter ounce at a time initially. Your output will rapidly improve as you get more skilled in the mechanics of pumping, your let-down gets conditioned to the pumping experience, and you become less anxious about your ability to express enough milk. To improve your chances of early success, try pumping when your breasts are full before your baby nurses. The shower is a good place to practice hand expression.

When you return to work, you will have to figure out when you will pump and, if not at home, where you will pump. Women have developed a variety of solutions to these problems. Many mothers who pump at work tried to pump at the times their babies would normally be nursing. For others the primary consideration was when they could take breaks from work with the least hassle so they could most easily relax to pump. In either case, it is important to develop a consistent schedule so your body will produce milk at regular times. An erratic schedule may cause your milk supply to dwindle.

Some of the pumping routines women have developed are summarized below. They may help you arrange a system that works for you.

Jackie Robbins, who returned to work full-time when her daughter was two months old, nursed her baby from the same breast at 4 and 7 A.M., then pumped from the other breast as soon as she got to work. She pumped a second time each day around 2 P.M. She went into her office and locked the door for privacy.

Sharon Martin, who returned to work full-time when her daughter was three months old, pumped twice a day, at ten and two, in the health unit of her office building. She went into a small cubicle with a cot and shut the door. Although it had initially taken her forty minutes to express three ounces while practicing at home, she had become skilled with the hand pump she used. Pumping took her ten minutes per side by the time she returned to work. She found that massaging her breast down toward the nipple while she pumped increased her efficiency.

Tina Horwitz, a second grade teacher, returned to work when Adam was almost four months old. She had no intention of pumping during the day, so she tried Adam on different formulas before her date to return. But he seemed to get stomachaches and be very gassy on formula, so she decided to pump. Tina pumped once a day at work at lunchtime. She had a planning session just before the lunch hour during which she would eat a sandwich she brought from home. She said,

I would eat quickly, then pump. It took me a few days to find a good place to do it. First I tried the health office but decided that would not do because kids were in and out all the time. Then I asked myself, "Where would *I* be most comfortable?" I didn't want to be nervous, and I didn't want anyone to barge in. My own classroom seemed like the best place. Since it was lunchtime, I knew where all the kids were, so I locked the door and sat sort of behind a file cabinet. It worked perfectly. At first I'd get about one or two ounces, but within a couple of weeks I was getting eight ounces in about twenty minutes.

When Maria Acevedo returned to work, she had trouble finding a place to pump. She worked in a laboratory with glass walls and no offices. The only place she could find privacy was in a bathroom stall, so that is where she pumped. Maria always felt a tingling in her breasts at the times when she would have nursed her son, so she pumped then. She always tried to pump one extra time during the day—one more time than her son was being fed at the sitter's. Her routine evolved into splitting her lunch hour into four fifteen-minute pumping breaks a day. She would get about four to six ounces each time.

Some women we met felt their jobs did not allow them the freedom to pump during the day. They could not be away from their desks for regular pumping sessions or there were no facilities for keeping the milk cold. It may be possible to overcome these limitations by trying to lay the groundwork ahead of time. One woman who was a secretary asked her boss if she could take two twenty-minute breaks a day for pumping and shorten her lunch hour. The boss agreed. You can ask your pediatrician to write a letter to your employer explaining the importance of your continuing to breastfeed your baby and asking him to provide you a pumping break. One woman arranged to store her pumped milk in a refrigerator in her building's cafeteria. You might experiment with a small styrofoam ice chest and freezer pack. Nonetheless, your job may not adapt to pumping. You may want or have to leave formula during the day.

Before You Return to Work

If you wish to leave breastmilk while you are away at work, you need to begin to practice pumping while you're still primarily at home. Here are some guidelines to help you get started.

• Practice pumping before you return to work to develop the skill necessary to express breastmilk efficiently. Try manual expression or choose a good pump. The Loyd-B seems especially popular among working mothers because of its transportability and use of baby food jars for collection. It takes some practice to master its use, but it is not too difficult for experienced nursing mothers. Chapter 4 discusses pumps in more detail.

• Moisten your breasts with water before applying the pump. It will create a better seal.

• Apply the pump so your nipple is off center. If the nipple comes into contact with the side of the pump and is rubbed backward and forward during the pumping action, more prolactin will be produced and hence more milk.

• Try massaging your breast as you pump to increase your efficiency.

• Pump from one breast as your baby nurses from the other to take advantage of the let-down response while nursing.

• Pump early in the morning when your breasts are full.

• Use vitamin E oil on your nipples if they become sore. (If you are allergic to wheat, you will need synthetic vitamin E.)

• If possible, build up a stockpile of six to eight bottles in the freezer before returning to work. This will be your insurance for the days you pump less than usual or when your baby suddenly starts demanding more. It is recommended that you freeze four ounces of milk at a time. If you collect less than this during one pumping session, put it in the refrigerator. At the end of the day, combine your cooled milk in units of four ounces and freeze it. (Chapter 4 contains guidelines on storing milk.)

Once You've Returned to Work

Once you have returned to work, the following suggestions may help you manage to pump effectively.

• Find a place to pump where you feel comfortable and are free from interruptions.

• Try to avoid working on anything anxiety- or tension-producing just before you pump. Anxiety increases your levels of adrenalin, and this blocks oxytocin, which stimulates your let-down reflex. So save your safe, boring, routine work for just before pumpings.

• If you are having particular difficulty one day getting your milk to let down, try stimulating your nipples the way your husband does during lovemaking.

• If you have problems getting a let-down response in the midst of hectic work days, consider using Syntocinon spray, a synthetic oxytocin preparation prescribed by your doctor. One woman told us, "I find it to be miraculous—it's made *all* the difference in my being able to pump at work—a very pressured situation in which I otherwise had tremendous difficulty with let-down."

• Pump on a regular schedule so your body can continue to produce milk at regular times. When you miss a particular feeding or pumping session for two or three days, your body is likely to stop producing milk at that time. If your pumping schedule is erratic, your body is likely to produce less milk.

• Drink lots of fluids, eat well, and get as much rest as possible. If your milk supply suddenly dwindles, you may need more rest.

• Consider taking your baby to bed with you to nurse frequently at night to keep up your milk supply.

• For moral support, talk to a friend who has pumped or call La Leche League.

Getting It All Together

Combining motherhood and work outside the home presents an ongoing series of challenges to the women who attempt this task. Working is never the same once you have become a mother. The dull days at the office can be harder to take. More days than not you may want to postpone the final touches on your projects or skip the socializing after work to return home to your baby. You may be torn when you have to leave home in the morning, especially if your child cries as you go. Yet it can be satisfying to work with people you like and use the skills and education you've acquired, earning money for your family. If your child is well cared for, and you have the desire, support, flexibility, and endurance to persist, working outside the home can be a viable option. Nursing your baby can be a delicious contrast to the hectic workaday world. It also means your baby continues to receive the antibodies and nutritional benefits of breastmilk. Being a working-nursing mother can be a fulfilling occupation.

On the other hand, it can also be enormously demanding. Nursing clearly places extra requirements on a woman who has responsibilities beyond her home and family. If you find that breastfeeding adds too much pressure to your already demanding life, weaning may be an appropriate alternative. You have given your baby a healthy start through the breastmilk you have provided since birth. It may be time to move on.

Your family's world is expanding with your working. Different situations always require some change. Your responsibility is to decide what works best within the context of your new schedule. Making such decisions will require you to be flexible in your approach. You may choose to cut back on your breastfeeding; you may choose to give it up entirely. Chapter 10 may help you to consider the process of weaning, whenever you feel the time is right.

9

Marriage and Sex

*This sex thing is a closet
issue. If I had understood that
so many people had
difficulty—that it takes time to
resume a normal sex
life—then I wouldn't have
worried so much.*

—A NEW MOTHER

WHEN WE TOLD friends that we were working on a chapter that would describe sexual activity and the marriage relationship after the birth of a child, reactions were remarkably similar. The usual response was something like "Well, *that* should be a very short chapter!" The information we were able to gather through interviews conveys a similar message: sexual activity is likely to be less frequent, and time for the marriage is difficult to arrange during the postpartum months. Nonetheless, although sexual and marital activity, as you once knew it, may seem to consume fewer of your hours, you may be expending considerable time and energy worrying about the changes you are experiencing.

Both you and your husband may be wondering what the odds are that your marriage and your sex lives can successfully coexist with the demands of a baby and breastfeeding.

In the weeks and months after the birth of their son, Linda and

Paul Ryan experienced some measurable differences in their sex lives. Linda had been told that she and Paul should not have intercourse until she had a postpartum checkup, to be scheduled four weeks from Travis's birth. But Linda didn't feel confident leaving Travis with a baby-sitter, and she didn't go back to the obstetrician until six weeks postpartum. She explained, "We did not rush right home to resume our old sex lives. For one thing, I really wasn't feeling so good. It had taken the doctor several tries to find a diaphragm that fit properly, and I was quite sore afterwards. So Paul and I waited a few days. That first time we made love, it was not wonderful, but it *was* a beginning."

Linda and Paul already understood that sex might be different while Linda was nursing. For one thing, they had been told that Linda would probably produce less vaginal lubrication. Beyond that, they had learned in their childbirth classes that they could expect differences in Linda's interest (could be more, could be less), in Linda's responsiveness (again, more or less), and in the way each of them might feel about involving Linda's breasts in sex play. They had also heard that postpartum fatigue could play an enormous role in their sexual activity. Perhaps because they had some preparation, this couple did not seem to be too worried about their altered sex lives.

Linda feels that the breastfeeding relationship she has with Travis provides her with much physical affection and, as a result, she doesn't feel the need for as much physical attention from Paul. Paul seems to have a reduced interest in sex, although Linda describes him as more affectionate, both physically and verbally, than before the birth.

> Most of the time we're both pretty tired. Hugging and holding each other can feel awfully good—and can be enough. I know we don't have an exciting sex life right now, but we know that this, too, shall pass. We talk about it and even laugh about it. On two occasions we were both feeling romantic in the middle of the afternoon, but we didn't get very far before the baby woke up. Sometimes I feel like we're in an old Doris Day movie.

Linda believes that the physical changes in her body have an effect on her feelings about sex. "I'm used to being thin and flat-chested. Now I have these big, round boobs, and I'm hippy. I feel full. I just don't feel sexy this way. I'm very self-conscious about my body." Also, Linda finds the idea of wearing a bra to bed unappealing. "I don't wear it during lovemaking, but I feel kind of messy with the leaking. I sometimes think that both Paul and I are avoiding my breasts. They're not erotic any more; they're functional." Linda and Paul have had intercourse three times in the three months since Travis's birth.

When talking about Paul and sex, Linda does not speak positively about her body. But when she speaks about her new motherhood, there's a change. She speaks with pride and confidence about the success with which her body is performing. "I feel womanly and I'm in awe of being able to feed Travis. His body is growing and developing because of me. It's amazing how capable a woman's body can be. I take such pleasure in seeing how he enjoys nursing."

What about Paul? Is he left out? Linda said that she did worry that Paul might feel that way. She figured that if she got to feed the baby, it was important for Paul to do some other things for Travis. "But the other things didn't seem to be as much fun. It's all worked out, though. Paul has always been the one who bathes the baby. They truly enjoy each other. I know that Paul feels good about my nursing. He looks on us with great pride. There's really enough love here to go around."

Resuming Sexual Intercourse

Women are usually advised to abstain from sexual intercourse for a period of time after childbirth to avoid infection while the uterus and episiotomy or tears (if there were any) are healing. In the course of our interviews, we learned that the advice given to women varies. Some doctors are still scheduling postpartum checkups six weeks after birth and advising mothers to have no sexual intercourse until after that checkup. Other doctors and nurse-midwives recommend only four weeks of abstinence. Still others instruct mothers to avoid sexual intercourse until the lochia (the bloody discharge from the uterus) subsides. This may take only two to three weeks, especially for mothers who are nursing frequently.

The directions given to the new mother should be specific, yet some practitioners simply remind women that, for two or four or six weeks, they are to have "no sex." The specific recommendation is for "no sexual intercourse." You may still be kissed and stroked and massaged and even brought to orgasm as long as nothing enters the vagina. Likewise, you are free to engage in sexual activity that brings your husband to orgasm. In the weeks after childbirth, affection, physical pleasure, and some sexual activity can be very important to the new parents. Avoiding sexual intercourse still can leave a pleasant range of possibilities.

Our interviews also showed that couples responded differently to the issue of sex in the early weeks. Some women noticed that they were anxious to resume sexual relations. Cynthia Pajak, a new mother who was on a three-month maternity leave, told us,

> My doctor said we had to wait till my six-week checkup. I was breast-feeding frequently, and my bleeding had stopped at ten days, and I thought we should be able to try it. Whenever I'd ask Tom what he thought, he'd say he wasn't a gynecologist and we should probably follow orders. Then, in a mothers' postpartum group, I discovered that other doctors only required four weeks of no sex. I told Tom, and that night we made love. We were just following a different doctor's orders!

On the other hand, Cynthia's neighbor, also a first-time mother, had strong negative feelings about resuming sex. "I've been for my four-week checkup. My doctor says it's okay to have sex now. Well, it's *not* okay with me! I wish I had a doctor who said six weeks. My sex drive has really dropped off."

There are some women who found that, though they were not particularly interested in sex itself, they wanted to recapture a sense of closeness to their husbands. These women seemed motivated by a desire for intimacy, and sex was important in helping them achieve it. One mother explained,

> In those first weeks, I was not really nice to be around. We weren't having sex. Mike had started running every night after work. We were very separate. That first Saturday after we had made love the night before, we sat at the kitchen table and talked about our bills . . . it was like old times. Our relationship is better since we started up sex again. We were distant before. Now we're talking again. And Mike even seems more interested in the baby.

For many couples, a return to sexual intimacy is not automatically a return to sex as they remember it. Elaine Duncan described her impression of postpartum lovemaking: "We made love at three weeks. It felt different from pregnant sex. My body felt different—it was a different shape, and we had gotten used to the feeling of a pregnant body. It was good, though. Jack said so, too. I felt relieved at that."

For other couples, sex after childbirth is more than "different." One woman explained, *"I* really wanted it. I wanted to be a sexy pre-pregnant woman again. My doctor said we could do it in two weeks if my bleeding had stopped. So we did. It was so unpleasant that we didn't do it again for another month!" Another mother described a similar experience: "We decided to try it. It was such a flop that we avoided sex for the next couple of weeks. You can tell you've got problems when you start doing Lamaze breathing to get through intercourse!"

Practical Considerations

There are several factors that can contribute to less-than-euphoric sex after childbirth. Besides the major issue of fatigue (which we'll discuss later), there are the following: (1) changes in your breasts and an altered body image; (2) discomfort during intercourse; and (3) birth control methods.

Changes in Your Breasts

While you are a nursing mother, you may notice some changes in your breasts that involve sex. Tender breasts and leaking milk were two concerns of some of the women we interviewed. One mother explained, "For me, it's distracting to have him touch my breasts. It hurts if my breasts are full, or if he's on top of me. Also, I worry about milk coming out."

The tenderness experienced in the early weeks or months of breastfeeding usually subsides or disappears as nursing progresses. For some mothers, it's the timing of sexual activity that makes a difference. "If I've just fed the baby, then it's okay. If there's a feeding coming up soon, then my breasts are too tender and it's not sexual." Some women are able to reduce the tenderness—what one woman called a feeling of "bruised boobs"—by expressing some milk (often in a warm shower) before lovemaking.

Many breastfeeding mothers notice that milk will leak from their breasts during sexual excitement. Women's reactions to this phenomenon differed. "I always had sex with my bra on and nursing pads inside the bra, because I didn't like the mess of leaking . . . and I felt that leaking milk would interfere with the mood." Another woman felt that *wearing* a bra interfered with the mood and so she took it off to make love. A towel on the bed kept the sheets dry. "I really didn't think it was such a big deal. I figured I was just wet somewhere else."

Although tenderness and leaking may cause some concern, for a number of nursing mothers the major change is increased breast size. Some women think that having larger breasts is terrific. "I love having breasts. I always wondered what it would be like." Other women are bothered by the increased size. "For months I looked forward to sleeping on my stomach, but I still can't because of the size of my breasts. I don't feel right with them." For the majority of women who experience a change in breast size, the reaction is one of ambivalence. Martha Goldsmith explained her feelings: "I don't feel uncomfortable physically. I feel psychologically uncomfortable. I *do* like the way I look in clothes, now. And it's nice to see how the other half lives, but I feel a little self-conscious. I was always small-chested, and now it's like I'm impersonating a woman."

For some women, like Linda in the beginning of this chapter, the ambivalence has much to do with the two roles they envision for their bodies. On one hand, the breastfeeding mother wants to nourish and nurture her baby; on the other, the new mother also wants a relationship with her husband. She would like to feel physically comfortable with him. She would like to believe that he finds her attractive and desirable. One mother of a four-month-old daughter explained her ambivalence:

> During the daytime, I feel proud. I was working in the yard the other day with Carrie in the back-pack. I looked down and noticed my large breasts, and I thought, "I'm strong. I'm carrying my baby, tending a garden. I have a good, capable, mothering body. I feel good." Then my husband comes home, and I feel self-conscious about my nursing body . . . it's not the body he married. He married a skinny woman with almost no boobs, but at least they were boobs he could use. Now I have these jugs that I don't want him to touch. In my mind, this mother's body doesn't work with him.

The dichotomy is clear. These women speak with pride when they consider their bodies in relation to their babies. But they talk about feeling self-conscious, embarrassed, or awkward about their bodies in relation to their husbands. Part of the problem may lie with a woman's difficulty in seeing or accepting her new role—mother—as a sexual one. ("Are mothers sexy?") The increased size of her breasts may remind the woman, more than any other bodily change, that she has become a nurturing, motherly female. Could this—does this—appeal sexually to her husband? Can the woman reconcile the roles of nurturer and lover?

Certainly there is plenty of suggestion in the media that large, round breasts are sexually appealing to men. For some nursing women, however, the difference between their breasts and the ones on television or in magazines is too clear. As one woman remarked, "The message you get is that breasts are supposed to be ornamental.

Those women [in the ads] have big breasts, but they're not full of milk." Another woman commented similarly about her breasts: "They're for work, not for decoration."

One of the challenges a woman may face as she becomes a breastfeeding mother is that of reconciling the dual roles of her breasts. As she begins to accomplish this, she may be better able to appreciate that her breasts can be both ornamental and functional, a source of both nourishment and sexual pleasure.

Something that might interfere temporarily with a woman's acceptance of her nursing body is the assumption so many of us had toward the end of pregnancy: "After I deliver this baby, I'll have my old body back again!" So we deliver our babies and . . . we *don't* have our old bodies back again! We have moved from pregnancy to lactation, with whatever alterations that may mean for our individual bodies. For those who had not been prepared for this next bodily adjustment, there may be some temporary sense of resentment or disappointment as the reunion with the old, familiar body is postponed even further.

Accepting the progression that the female body makes from conception through pregnancy, lactation, and weaning—and seeing it as valuable and logical—may help to improve your feelings about your body. One first-time mother seemed to have no trouble accepting these physical changes because they made sense to her. "My breasts didn't get big overnight. They grew with my pregnancy and just stayed around for a while. It's like I got them for the occasion."

Some women who initially feel self-conscious about their changed bodies find that their awkwardness diminishes as the weeks and months go by. (It's also possible that the fullness of their breasts decreases over the months. This is not because of diminished milk supply but because of adjustments the body makes over time.) The fuller body that, at first, seemed unfamiliar becomes more comfortable and acceptable. The new mother can begin to appreciate her nursing body not just because it can sustain her child but also because her healthy female body is capable of giving and receiving both sensual and sexual pleasure. As time passes, some women begin to notice that the increased size of their breasts makes them feel more erotic during sex play. As one woman said, "I feel better in a way. When we're making love, it's like I bring more to it."

Men also may have some initial reservations about the changes in their wives' bodies. Some women find, however, that their husbands are flattering and appreciative. It seems important not to make assumptions about what your husband is thinking and feeling. A number of women who spoke candidly to us had never conversed with their spouses about postpartum sex. Nonetheless, most of these women were prepared to make assumptions—to guess—about their husbands' reactions.

> I can tell he's avoiding my breasts. He's probably afraid of hurting me.

> He hasn't commented at all. If he liked the difference, I guess he'd say so.

> He thinks my larger breasts are great. He caresses them and kisses them, but not near the nipple part. Maybe he thinks that's for the baby . . . or maybe he doesn't want to get any milk.

Each marriage develops its own style. Some couples seem to be more comfortable avoiding discussions of intimate topics. But if silence in this area begins to cause confusion, awkwardness, and hurt feelings, it may mean that the time has come to explore—to whatever degree seems comfortable or agreeable—each partner's concerns and feelings. The following are examples of how behavior—without discussion or explanation—can be misinterpreted.

> She: "I think the idea of milk in my breasts sort of disgusts him. He won't put his mouth near my nipples."
> He: "I think it's a bad idea to suck on her nipples. What about the baby getting my germs? What about getting milk that's supposed to be for the baby?"

She: "I feel like I'm schizophrenic. I don't want him handling my breasts, but then when he doesn't I think, 'Why isn't he interested in my breasts anymore?' "

He: "She's been through so much and she's doing so much for the baby now. When it comes to sex, I don't want to press. She must get tired of everyone—the baby and me—wanting her body for something."

Sex and the breasts of a nursing mother . . . what does *she* think? What does *he* think? Predictably, feelings and behavior vary from person to person, from couple to couple.

Of the women we interviewed, many did not enjoy having their breasts handled during sex.

I think I give out the message, "Don't mess with my breasts." I feel very protective of them.

My breasts used to be erotic. Now I see them as a source of the baby's food. Maybe that's how he sees them, too. They're not included in sex play as much as they used to be.

I don't care to have my breasts fondled by him. They're really zoned out while I'm nursing.

On the other hand, some women find that they experience a heightened sensitivity in their nipples and breasts which enhances their sexual feelings. One mother explained, "After having a baby at my breasts all day, I find I can be rather interested in some adult activity. I feel very responsive when my husband strokes or sucks my breasts." Among some couples, the nursing mother's breasts are accepted comfortably as both useful for the baby and pleasurable for the parents. One mother described her husband's occasional reaction: "Sometimes when I'm nursing on the bed, he'll kiss my breast and then kiss the baby."

Whether a couple avoids or enjoys sexual activity that involves the woman's breasts, the more important consideration may be whether they both agree. One mother of a three-month-old son told us that she had looked forward to experiencing sex as a nursing mother because of a novel she had read. She recalled the descriptive sex scenes and the pleasure the man felt making love to his nursing lover. Her own experience was different. When she encouraged her husband to taste her milk, he refused. "He just won't do it. He has made it clear that he doesn't intend to mix milk with sex!"

Through our interviews we learned that some couples change their attitudes as time passes. They may react differently as the months go by, or as they progress from the first child to the second child. One thirty-five-year-old father explained his feelings about sucking on his wife's breasts: "I thought it was bad because I'd be taking the milk. It was some time before I learned that the more sucking there is, the more milk there is. Then I no longer felt I was 'competing.'"

A father of two daughters described his gradual change of attitude: "When we first had a baby, a colleague at work asked if I had tasted breastmilk yet. I was appalled! Of course not! What kind of pervert was he? Now after two children, I must say I've tasted breastmilk often. It's not as good as a vodka and tonic, but I certainly don't think it's perverted anymore."

Some men spoke of "getting over the inhibition," and some men explained that they just couldn't. "It wasn't my territory. I shouldn't be there." One father of three older children thinks that if he were to do it all again, he might react differently. "But at the time, I was repulsed. I'd think, 'I'm thirty years old and I'm sucking a mother's nipples.' I just didn't think it through."

Women, too, spoke of changes in attitude. A mother of three children told us that her feelings differed from one child to the next. "When I was nursing our first, I enjoyed having my breasts included in sex play. With the second child, I didn't. With the third, I enjoyed it again. I have no idea why it was different each time." Another woman explained that she needed time to adjust to the changes in her body: "Our baby was about three months old before I got used to my nursing body and considered my breasts erotic. When I finished weaning her at nine months, my breasts got small again. I remember feeling self-conscious. I had gotten used to fuller breasts. It probably took me another month to feel comfortable with my smaller size."

Discomfort during Intercourse

After childbirth, you might experience some discomfort during intercourse. For one thing, there are hormonal changes taking place in your body that can cause you to lubricate less during sexual activity. The resulting vaginal dryness can make intercourse most uncomfortable. (This is true whether you have a vaginal birth or a Cesarean birth.) Women who are breastfeeding are likely to experience this reduced lubrication for a longer period of time. Some form of lubrication (K-Y jelly, for example, or contraceptive cream) can be used during foreplay to make penetration more comfortable. (Avoid petroleum jelly because it is not water-soluble and because, over time, it can cause damage to the latex of diaphragms.)

Another cause of painful intercourse might be an episiotomy or a tear that is healing. Because of the location of your stitches, it might be necessary for you and your partner to try different positions in lovemaking. Pressure should be shifted away from the back of the vagina (where the stitches are located) and toward the front (in the direction of the clitoris). This may be most easily accomplished by the woman being on top of her husband during intercourse.

If you are very tense during intercourse, penetration can be uncomfortable. You may benefit from a hot bath (if bleeding has stopped) or a shower before making love. The relaxation techniques you learned for childbirth can be useful to you now. Notice where your body is tense and try to relax those muscles. Notice your breathing and allow it to be slow and deep and rhythmic. Try to be patient with yourself. And explain your concerns to your husband, so that he won't have to guess what's going on. "In the beginning, I thought I was stitched up wrong. I felt that intercourse would be impossible. And I think I gave my husband the impression that I wasn't interested . . . that he just couldn't get me excited."

It might be useful for you to view your first postpartum attempt at sex as strictly exploratory. You both may feel less worried about the outcome if you decide ahead of time that "this one won't count." One woman explained that she felt less pressure to perform or respond because they had agreed to this. "I was very sensitive. The first time we didn't even expect to finish. Penetration was enough."

If, after taking appropriate measures (for lubrication, position, and relaxation), you continue to hurt during intercourse as the weeks go by, you should consult your doctor or nurse-midwife. He or she might want to examine you again. In some cases, a prescribed salve can help.

Birth Control

Unrestricted breastfeeding (no supplementary bottles, frequent nursings day and night, and limited or no use of pacifiers) appears to be very effective in suppressing ovulation, but it is not a guarantee. Therefore, if you don't want to get pregnant, you need to choose some form of birth control.

Women who breastfeed should avoid the pill. The high concentration of hormones present in the pill can pass through your milk and be ingested by your baby. If you plan to have an IUD inserted (if they are still on the market), you must wait until you are eight weeks postpartum, according to a Food and Drug Administration regulation. It is important that your uterus has involuted (shrunk down) to a nonpregnant state so that the chance of infection and perforation is reduced. Similarly, if you choose to use the diaphragm or a cervical sponge, you need to wait until your uterus has returned to its nonpregnant size. If you are nursing without restrictions, this involution might occur in four weeks. Otherwise, it can take at least six weeks. It is at this point that your doctor or nurse-midwife can fit you for a diaphragm. (If you used a diaphragm before you got pregnant, that same diaphragm may not be the right size for you now. Have the fit checked by your doctor or nurse-midwife.)

While you are waiting to use the IUD, diaphragm, or sponge,

or to go on the pill, you can use condoms and foam for birth control. It is often recommended that you use *both* to increase the effectiveness of each method. Some couples choose to avoid the pill and the IUD because of health considerations and continue the practice of condoms and foam. Others find condoms alone to be effective.

The possibility of a new pregnancy can be an overwhelming consideration for some couples. In the early weeks before being able to use a diaphragm, one nursing mother found that she could not bring herself to have intercourse using condoms and foam: "I didn't care what the statistics were. I would not take a chance on getting pregnant."

There's another problem regarding birth control methods. For couples who were accustomed to a method that required no on-the-spot preparation, the options now available can have some effect on their sexual activity. One woman explained that, when first married, she had used the pill. She went off the pill and eventually got pregnant. During pregnancy, sex was pleasurable and no issue. After almost five years of either the pill or no birth control, she was now using the diaphragm. She found this new method bothersome and believed it contributed to less frequent sex.

Whichever method of birth control you and your husband choose, it is likely that it will involve some trade-offs. The pill and the IUD are less bothersome at the time of lovemaking, but both methods are subjects of concern regarding a woman's health. The diaphragm, cervical sponge, or condoms and foam are safer for the mother, but they are considered by many to reduce spontaneity, romance, and physical pleasure. If you choose one of these less convenient methods, you need to acknowledge the effect it might have on your sexual activity. You may find that sexual spontaneity is more difficult with the birth control method you've chosen. You and your husband will benefit from talking about your concerns. You need to be patient with yourselves and your bodies. This is a time of adjustment. It will help if you occasionally can muster up a sense of humor about the whole thing, remember you like each other, remember how nice sex *can* be for the two of you, and proceed with the confidence that things *will get better.*

Frequency (or Infrequency) of Sex

For many new parents, sex is less frequent than before. Although some couples may be able to pick up right where they left off, most of the people we spoke to reported noticeable differences in sex after the birth of a child. For some couples, the differences lasted only a few months; for others, the changes were obvious at least throughout the first year. All couples seemed to have a sense of having been unprepared for the changes. As the mother of an eight-month-old told us,

> I was so afraid that I would never feel sexual again. I found it difficult to get excited. I remember that when our childbirth instructor said it takes a while for your sex lives to adjust, I thought she meant *weeks*, so I started to worry as the months went by. When I talked to her later, she said the adjustment might be gradual over the first year. It certainly would have helped me to know that.

Another new mother expressed similar feelings: "This sex thing is a closet issue. If I had understood that so many people had difficulty—that it takes time to resume a normal sex life—then I wouldn't have worried so much."

There are several reasons for a decrease in sexual activity after the birth of a child. The increased fatigue generally felt by new parents can have an impact. Balancing your needs for sexual intimacy with an often overwhelming requirement for rest is extremely difficult. Additionally, there is likely to be a lessening in frequency as you move from spontaneous to planned lovemaking. There is also some evidence that both men and women may experience reduced sexual energy during the postpartum months. Clearly, adjustments in the sexual area are in order, and a positive attitude—and a sense of humor—can help.

Fatigue

Since bottle-feeding mothers may also experience less frequent sex, there must be something beyond the specifics of nursing

that contributes to this phenomenon. Whether a baby is breastfed or
bottle-fed, the mother and father of an infant are frequently too tired
for sex. A mother of three children expressed her feelings: "We're
both experiencing fatigue. This may be nature's way of family planning. There usually seem to be more reasons *not* to have sex than
to have it. It has happened after the births of all three children, but
it's less of an issue each time." As another woman explained, "Even
before we had a baby, being tired affected our sex lives. This is
nothing new, it's just that we're tired more often now."

One woman we interviewed explained that, though she generally felt too tired for sex, she was annoyed that there was not more
physical affection between her and her husband. "It can't just be sex
or nothing." It is important that new parents communicate with each
other verbally and physically. If a new father understands that his
wife is too tired or disinterested in sex and if he believes that his
displays of affection will be interpreted as "overtures" to sex, he may
not feel comfortable being physically affectionate toward her. "I
don't want her to think that after satisfying the baby all day long she
should have to think about satisfying me."

The man and woman who can talk to each other about their
feelings will find that they may become more relaxed and reassured
about what's happening to them. Couples who express their concerns to each other often report a sense of "being in this thing
together." They have to worry less about being misinterpreted (always a likely possibility where sex is concerned), and they conserve
energy often wasted on mind-reading (sometimes irresistible but
generally inaccurate).

Some new parents find that, though they have very little energy
for full-fledged sex, they need and enjoy some physical intimacy. A
woman who had recently given birth to her second child explained,
"The frequency and duration of lovemaking are different for us
now. There is a tenderness. Just touching each other and kissing and
being together is nice. It doesn't have to culminate in sex. And he
doesn't act as if he's being denied or cheated."

One woman commented on a difference in her husband since
their baby's birth: "Rob is much more affectionate. He's softer,
demonstrative, different." Another new mother had a similar obser-

vation about her husband: "Al has learned new ways to demonstrate affection because we can't count on the same old way." It seems crucial that the new mother be willing to recognize and accept new expressions or demonstrations of affection. Her husband may call from work during the day to see how things are going; when he's home he might take over some child care so she can shower or nap; when she sits down to nurse the baby he might bring her something to drink. It would be sad for both of them if she didn't recognize such activities as expressions of affection.

Verbal affection can sometimes help to fill the void created by infrequent sex. One woman described an evening when she and her husband had been particularly compatible and relaxed together. Before they were able to get to bed, however, the baby woke, nursed at length, and required a considerable amount of rocking and walking before he went back to sleep. "I was feeling a little cheated. Like, would we have had sex if things had been different? I felt better when I got into bed and Mike said, 'I'd really like to make love to you, but I'm so tired now.' It was really important that he told me."

The verbal affection may not even have anything to do with sex. In the early weeks after their baby's birth, one father occasionally woke during night feedings and would sleepily remark to his wife: "Thanks for feeding the baby." Another woman remarked: "Sometimes, when Gordon says something nice to me, like about how I'm good with the baby or how well the nursing seems to be going . . . well, I almost feel caressed."

Planning Opportunities

Although the complications of breastfeeding and increased fatigue may be responsible for some changes in sexual activity, there is another issue. New parents may experience less frequent sex because it is difficult to arrange for *more* frequent sex. "Our schedules are so crazy. It's hard to fit sex in. It's been four weeks now, and I guess we should probably do it. Henry says whenever I'm ready . . . as long as it's not next year."

With the demands of an infant, a home, jobs, grocery shopping, friends and relatives, and the need for sleep, it can be most difficult to find both the energy and the time for sex. This is easy to understand as a logical matter, but it can still be troublesome. The nagging questions can keep forcing their way into your consciousness. You know there's no time, but if you *really* loved each other, wouldn't you *find* the time? Shouldn't your sexual lives take priority over some other demands? Does this mark the beginning of a mediocre sex life? One woman explained her thinking during the first six or seven months: "One thought gave me the most difficulty: is this to be expected, or is there something going seriously wrong and I'm not realizing it?"

Suddenly there is a need to create opportunities. For many couples, the arrival of children marks the beginning of a period of planned sex. "We used to be such spontaneous people. Now we have to set a date for having sex." The plans for sexual intimacy vary. One couple arranged to get into bed on Sunday afternoons when their daughter was napping. Another couple set aside Friday nights. "Maybe it sounds contrived, but it worked out well for us. On Friday I knew I had to get ready for our 'date.' I would plan dinner, take a shower, wash my hair. It was just better for us to plan."

One woman, whose baby woke frequently during the night and slept very little during the day, described their routine: "Sometimes in the evening Paul takes the baby so that I can nap. If I can get that little extra sleep, I can be much more responsive." Another couple doesn't share the same bed during the week because of their wakeful baby. Dad sleeps in the guestroom. The mother told us, "For about an hour at bedtime we all get in the same bed. There's a chance for Bob and me to talk and cuddle. Sex is saved for the weekends, usually afternoons. We're both very busy and tired during the week. Actually, it was often like that even before the baby. We know we have to plan for sex now—put it in our schedule."

Of course, planning an opportunity for lovemaking does not guarantee it. The baby may not be a cooperative party to your plans. Even the *possibility* of the baby's waking can interfere. One mother explained: "The big question is how to find a good time for making love. I always have one ear cocked. I hear a sound. I freeze. Is he waking up?" One woman remarked: "We're snuggling less. I'd rather do nothing than be interrupted. We just don't get started."

Several mothers mentioned the need to set aside enough time to relax and allow for the possibility of making love. As one mother explained, "It seems like it takes me longer to get in the mood. Every time we start lovemaking, I feel like saying 'Wait a minute. . . . Wait a minute. . . . I'm not ready.' " Some couples recognize this need and make appropriate arrangements. "If we are interested in sex, we go to bed at nine, so there'll be time to talk."

Interest Level

In their book *Human Sexual Response,* William Masters and Virginia Johnson report that nursing mothers express a greater sexual interest in the first three months after childbirth than nonnursing mothers. The nursing mothers reported being interested in resuming sexual intercourse with their husbands as soon as possible. This bit of information is often used to suggest that women who are breastfeeding are likely to be more sexually active. This is an inaccurate reading of their findings. Masters and Johnson meant exactly what they said. The nursing mothers they interviewed were *interested* in sexual activity. No information was collected regarding actual performance.

In the course of a normal day, a nursing mother may feel particularly interested in sex at two o'clock in the afternoon. Perhaps she has just nursed the baby. The baby has fallen asleep. The house is quiet. She has time to take a shower and wash her hair. She is feeling relaxed, serene, and sexy. Her husband is at work. If anyone is keeping score, that amounts to interest, 1; performance, 0.

As the day progresses, it is not uncommon for both mother and baby to deteriorate. Eleven o'clock at night becomes an unacceptable time to do something about her two o'clock interest. As one mother explained, "My husband and I have access to each other at the worst time of the day."

Although some nursing mothers report increased feelings of sexuality, others claim that their interest in sex was reduced. One woman said, "I feel affectionate but not sexy." Another explained, "I feel compliant but not particularly interested."

It is possible that breastfeeding is partly responsible for reduced libido. It may be that hormonal activity during lactation has an impact on sexuality. It may be that the nursing relationship diminishes a woman's desire for sex.

Many women made similar observations about their reduced sexual activity. "I think breastfeeding interferes. I have a physical relationship with the baby and I find that I don't crave one with my husband." Another woman agreed: "My husband needed sex more than I did in the first eight or nine months. He wasn't getting the gratification I was getting—the hugging and the coziness—all day." This imbalance in the marital relationship can be confusing and disturbing.

For some women, the issue is one of limitations. They feel as though the breastfeeding relationship leaves very little room for other intimate activity. "I feel I can only handle one thing at a time. Right now my body mostly belongs to the baby." A woman who recently gave birth to her second child explained her reactions: "My husband is very interested in sex. When he starts making overtures, I start thinking, 'I'm going to be consumed. I'm going over the edge.' He doesn't remember that it was like this after our first child. I'm good at one-on-one relationships. Nursing definitely complicates my relationship with him."

This alteration in your sexual interest or responsiveness can be disturbing to both you and your husband, but it does not represent a permanent change. It is true that even twelve months after birth many couples report that frequency of sex hasn't returned to the rate of prebaby days, but many do claim that, season by season, their sex lives improve. One new father, who listened to a discussion of this issue, tried to put things into perspective: "When I was holding down two jobs, sex was less frequent. When I was working and going back to school, sex was less frequent. This is not the first time we've gone through a period like this, and it probably won't be the last. This is just the way life and sex go."

Adjusting

The couples who seem to be functioning best with the changes in their sex lives are the ones who are willing to make some adjustments in their expectations. They do not equate reduced sexual interest during the postpartum months with a deteriorating marriage. They recognize many of the changes in their relationship as normal, logical, and inevitable. Marriage with a child is different than marriage without a child. Wendy Yoder, a first-time mother, reflected on some of the changes:

> It's difficult if you expect the same kind of sex life as before. If you still try to live that other life, there are problems. You have to change what you think of as romantic. I used to associate sex with having a really nice date with Neil. Now we take walks together. Neil carries the baby in the front-pack. I like to look at them together and think about how Neil and I created that little baby. Or we'll splurge and buy a steak. While I nurse the baby, Neil cuts my meat, and I feel good that together we're managing. We're a team.

It may help to create new definitions of romance, as this woman did, since much of the romance of your prebaby days might be difficult to experience right now. Did it involve dinner out, a movie, stimulating conversation, lazy mornings, a day of outdoor exercise, a clean house, sexy clothes? The problem is not so much diminishing romantic interest in your partner. It is more the lack of opportunities to allow that interest to surface. One new mother remarked: "Think of what you were like—and what your life was like—at the peak of your sexual life. How much of your life is like that now?" And while you are discovering new situations that may seem romantic to you,

you may also need to reassess your feelings about sex and a successful marriage. One woman suggested that the changes in her sex life would have been easier to live with if it weren't for the flood of discussions in the media about sex. "It's as if all of society is hung up on sex and can't go forty-eight hours without it." The success of a marriage, the closeness of the partners, cannot be measured by the number of times they make love each month. Even before having children, many couples could describe periods of increased and decreased passion.

Throughout your life you experience changes in your sex life. Some weeks, some seasons, are more sexually exciting and fulfilling than others. It's important not to panic if sex is, at the moment, infrequent or unappealing or without passion. Many of us can't have "all systems go" with any degree of effectiveness. While you are learning to love a new child, to adjust to yourself as a mother, to accept responsibility for breastfeeding and child care, it's understandable if sex is not one of your strong points.

The couples who see themselves as "going through a phase" in their postpartum sex lives seem better able to cope with the alterations. Those couples who are able to express their concerns and tolerate their differences, who are willing to arrange for new lovemaking opportunities and to accept affection and romance in new forms will probably experience less anxiety.

⁓ 10 ⁓

Weaning

*Parenting doesn't stop with
weaning . . . I thought of this
as I set the table tonight with
one less dish than last night.
Our college boy went back to
school after a weekend at
home. The feeling I had was
much like the twinge I felt at
the weaning of my nursling.*

—MARIE-BERNICE DOWNEY,
Virginia Visions

ALTHOUGH the issue of weaning is a theme that runs
throughout the nursing experience, at some times it seems more
important than at others. One of the most common questions posed
by new nursing mothers is "How long should I breastfeed?" In the
early days of nursing, mothers may frequently contemplate weaning
as they wonder whether they can manage breastfeeding at all. They
also may question how long they'll be able to remain committed to
such an all-consuming job. As one mother explained, "I began to
think about weaning right after my baby was born. But soon the
overwhelming aspects of nursing faded away and breastfeeding became integrated into the rest of my life."

Once nursing is established and is no longer a project in its own right, the need to know when it will end seems to diminish. Except for the occasional bad day, when weaning is contemplated as the solution for all sorts of ailments or when the mother feels pressure from others, the middle period of nursing is usually free of concerns about weaning.

There comes a time, however, when the question of weaning reemerges. Either the mother or the child begins to indicate that the time for nursing is coming to a close. As one mother said, "When Clementine began to walk, she could no longer be bothered to nurse." Another said, "Greg is six months old now and I feel myself ready to stop nursing him. I want to be able to leave him with a sitter. I'm beginning to feel confined. I'm sick of wearing nursing bras. I can't wear sundresses because they're not comfortable. I'm ready to wean." When signs of readiness appear, weaning becomes a serious issue again.

Weaning entails substituting cow's milk, formula, or food for breastmilk and technically begins as soon as the baby eats or drinks anything besides breastmilk. The process is begun with that first supplementary bottle or spoonful of cereal, even if the mother has no intention of ending breastfeeding at that time.

When mothers ask about weaning, however, their concern is usually about the end of the weaning process. "When will I no longer be breastfeeding? How will we get to that point?" Mothers question how they will gently bring to a close an experience that has been such an important part of their relationship with their child.

In this chapter we shall define weaning as the efforts to complete the nursing experience. This means the mother is intentionally providing a substitute for nursing. Her goal is to stop breastfeeding. Weaning does not, however, imply aggressiveness or speed. The weaning process should be accomplished gradually, gently, and lovingly.

When Ellen Dragsten's son Zach was twelve months old, she began looking for signs that he was ready to wean. He'd been drinking out of a cup since he was five and a half months old, and he was adept at it. "But," Ellen commented, "he showed no signs of losing interest in my breast. He had never been interested in a bottle, a pacifier, his thumb, or a blanket."

Ellen decided to try to encourage weaning by nursing only when Zach "asked" by pulling on her shirt. She gave him his solids early before his usual nursing times. She tried to distract him and interest him in other security objects. But nothing worked. Zach's interest in nursing did not seem to diminish. Then Ellen decided that if she wanted to begin weaning, she'd have to be more organized about it. "I decided then to make an effort to find a substitute for one nursing at a time. I could tell Zach wasn't going to stop yet without my help, and I was feeling ready to move on. I'd always imagined weaning him at about a year, and here we were beyond that and we hadn't even begun. I knew it would probably take us several months, so I wanted to begin."

At that time Zach and Ellen enjoyed going swimming together, so Ellen decided to use trips to the pool as a substitute for Zach's midmorning nursing. She planned to go each morning before Zach usually asked to nurse. Ellen said they made a ritual of having a juice and raisin snack at the pool, then staying there through lunch.

The first few days, Zach tried to open Ellen's beach robe as they left for the pool. Ellen responded by saying, "We're going to the pool, Zach. We'll nurse when we get home." She was surprised that he didn't protest strongly. Within about a week, Zach seemed to have forgotten about the morning nursing.

The next week Ellen substituted a story, cuddling, and juice for their late afternoon nursing. She observed that if she caught Zach before he asked to nurse, he could usually be held off until dinner. The afternoon routine included having juice with Zach, then rocking him and reading him a story. The first few days Zach tugged on Ellen's shirt as they read, and Ellen said, "Zach this is story time. Then we're going for a walk." Zach continued to show interest in nursing through the story. Ellen responded by holding him snugly and rocking as she tried to interest him in the book's pictures.

Ellen said she was amazed how readily Zach accepted substitutes for nursing once she was consistent about offering them. Their early morning nursing was more difficult to change, however. Since they always nursed in Ellen's bed before getting up for the day, she said she set her alarm to get up before he did. When it went off, she forced herself to get up, get dressed, and go to the kitchen to make breakfast. Her husband brought Zach down for breakfast as soon as Zach got up. "The first week I had trouble, though," confided Ellen. "Zach seemed so drowsy when he came to breakfast. He looked so little and vulnerable. I couldn't help holding him in my arms and nursing him on the couch. He seemed to need the quiet time together to start the day. I needed it, too," Ellen continued. She didn't go back to nursing him in bed, but they did nurse on the couch for a week or so.

When Zach was about fourteen months old and just nursing before his afternoon nap and at bedtime, Ellen slowed the weaning process for a while. "I felt we needed the rest from 'programs.' I had been so organized during those previous two months of weaning that I was tired of thinking about it. Besides I felt more relaxed about nursing. I knew now I could wean Zach. I knew it was possible."

When Ellen decided to get on with the weaning process, she did so by changing their bedtime routines. Instead of rocking Zach to sleep while nursing, Ellen began to lie down with him in her bed and rub his back until he fell asleep.

> Before we changed routines, I told him, "Mommy's milk is going away because you are getting bigger. You are not a little baby anymore." He cried one night while I rubbed his back and sang to him. After that, he didn't even ask for milk. It was so easy, I think he was ready. But I still lie down with him every night. I really enjoy being with him at bedtime. It's different than all the other parts of the day.

Ellen's story has introduced several of the issues that women face as they begin to consider and proceed through the process of weaning a child. In this chapter we shall discuss the decision to wean, including the ambivalence many mothers experience. We will also describe the process of weaning and the mother's and child's life after weaning.

The Decision to Wean

The decision to wean is not made lightheartedly by most women. Many contemplate the issue for a period of time. Mothers ask others about their experiences and try to assess whether they and their children are ready. Plans for weaning are made and changed; schedules for weaning are begun and dropped. This is not surprising since nursing means so much more than providing milk for your baby. Several factors seem to influence the decision to wean: pressure from others, the role nursing has played in your mothering, and how the question of timing affects your needs and your baby's needs.

It is possible that as nursing continues you will begin to sense that other people—perhaps relatives, friends, or even health care professionals—have definite ideas about how long you should nurse. Sometimes this interest becomes explicit pressure to wean. Regardless of *your* questions about weaning, other people may be sure the time has come. One mother found that the further her baby grew past the six-month mark, the faster came the questions about when she would wean. Outside pressure may also come in the form of disapproval of your plans to *stop* breastfeeding. Sometimes it is hard to resist the pressure. Don't hesitate to muster your resources by finding the support of someone who is sympathetic to your point of view. Your decisions about weaning should not have to please your neighborhood, colleagues, or in-laws.

Another factor that may influence you is the degree to which breastfeeding has become part of your style of mothering. Some mothers get so accustomed to nursing their children at particular times, such as bedtime, that it is hard to imagine managing those times without it. One mother of a ten-month-old said she was beginning to consider weaning but could not figure out how she would ever get her baby to sleep without nursing. Nursing may become embedded in your ways of calming your child, relaxing with him, cuddling him, and starting and ending your days with him. Thus weaning may mean changing a very basic ingredient in your relationship with each other. Taking on the responsibility for making that change can be difficult—especially if your child enjoys nursing.

The question of *when* to wean is one of the major considerations of a mother facing this decision. It usually includes judgments about the baby's readiness or capacity to give up nursing, as well as the mother's need or desire to end the breastfeeding experience.

Scientific knowledge can give us some insight into the question of the baby's physical readiness. Studies tell us that at six months the baby's gut becomes less permeable to foreign proteins, thus reducing the chance of allergies to cow's milk or solid food. By the end of the first year the sucking fat pads in the baby's cheeks begin to disappear so he can chew more efficiently. At about twenty-four months the baby's immunological system is mature enough to reduce the need for the antibodies provided by breastmilk. Yet science cannot tell us outright how long we should nurse. Even if science could provide that information, the motivation to nurse or wean is not based on facts alone. Each of us must decide when the time is right for us and our children.

Some mothers consciously choose not to wean their babies or toddlers until the child loses interest in nursing. La Leche League argues persuasively that our culture pressures women into weaning their babies far before the babies are ready. In many parts of the world children nurse well beyond their toddlerhood. And the evidence suggests that these children become very independent. Having had their needs for sucking, contact, and security adequately met through nursing, these children seem to be secure enough to move away from their mothers toward their siblings, their peers, and other significant adults.

In our society, mothers who choose to nurse for more than a year say they find little support in the community at large. In any case, it is important for you to know that many mothers do wait to wean until their baby begins the process. This has been called "baby-led" weaning. Some babies begin to lose interest in nursing at about nine months; for others it is much later. La Leche League offers excellent support and guidance for mothers who choose to follow their child's initiatives.

Other mothers find themselves interested in weaning before their babies have begun to wean themselves. This has been called "mother-led" weaning. At any one time there are probably a number of reasons both to continue and to stop nursing. Each of us weighs these factors periodically. We all have our own mental scales that attempt to balance our child's needs to nurse with the needs of ourselves and other family members for us not to nurse. Not nursing may mean more time, predictability, and freedom to engage in other pursuits.

Most of the mothers we met began weaning because they felt ready to do so. Whether their babies were two months old or two years old, most of these mothers seemed to have reached a point where they felt ready to wean *and* they felt their children could give up nursing. This maternal readiness was expressed in a number of ways.

One mother said that when her son was four months old, she was ready to have her body back to herself and be thin again. "I was so tired of the maternity clothes I was still wearing and of the big blouses that were best for nursing. I got to the point where I really wanted my freedom, and I wanted to diet." A mother of a seven-month-old said she wanted to wean because she had started to work outside her home. She found working and nursing exhausting, and she felt physically ready to stop nursing. Another mother decided to wean her son when he was twelve months old and she wanted to send him to a preschool program a couple of mornings a week. "I was going stir-crazy," she confided. "I felt we both needed the change."

Nonetheless, even when mothers had decided and were committed to weaning, many still reported feeling uncertain and uneasy in this new phase of mothering. No matter how ready or willing your baby appears to be to move on to the next stage, or how ready you are to get back to the life of a nonnursing woman, you may find you still have questions about your decision.

You may encounter this ambivalence because of the closeness and satisfaction you've experienced nursing your child. Weaning means that the specific physical relationship of breastfeeding, which may have offered you a pleasurable or gratifying way of feeding your baby, is soon to be over. It is not uncommon to feel some nostalgia for this early mothering experience.

Furthermore, weaning requires a mother to add a new dimension to her parenting role. You now will be denying your child something he may want and something you could give but have decided to withhold. This theme will recur over and over again throughout your parenthood. Your child will want something you've decided, for whatever reason, not to provide: more candy, a skateboard, use of the car. This can be one of the difficult and challenging aspects of parenting. Weaning may be your introduction to it.

Finally, your ambivalence may stem from your perception of your baby's needs in relation to your own. You may want to stop nursing to be free to work away from home but have doubts about whether your baby is ready for you to spend more time away. Or you may feel unsure of yourself simply because your child seems to enjoy nursing so much. Your concern may focus on how well your baby will be able to manage the weaning process and adjust to new routines.

As time passes, you and your child *will* move beyond nursing. Some mothers talk about having felt ambivalent about weaning for months—they felt the baby was getting old enough to wean yet sensed their own reluctance to begin the process. They may have even tried to wean halfheartedly for several months, not really believing it could or would be accomplished. But then, suddenly, the pieces fell into place and they felt sure it was time to complete the weaning process. One mother said she suddenly "psychologically weaned" her twelve-month-old daughter. Even though the actual completion of nursing took several more weeks, she knew from then on that weaning was best for her and acceptable for her daughter. Thus she continued the process with a feeling of resolve.

Although ambivalence can be distressing, it is probably useful. It gives you the time to consider each factor in your decision. It invites you to look at your child more closely and at yourself more honestly. It heightens your interest in figuring out what is going on with each of you. Being ambivalent about whether to begin weaning indicates how much you care about making the right decision.

Preparation for Weaning

As you begin to think about weaning, you can start to prepare for it.

• Become aware of your pattern of nursing. Observe which nursings are your child's least favorite. Notice whether nursing is attached to any regular activities such as your talking on the telephone or watching the evening news on television. Are you the one who usually offers to nurse without your child taking the initiative? If so, does this mean your child could be ready to give up some nursing?

• Watch for the periods when your child's interest in the world is expanding. Weaning is often easier when your child is absorbed with new activities than when he is feeling clingy and unsure of himself and his world. Some babies, however, seem to need to return to the security of nursing between bouts of bravery and exploration.

• You may find information which claims that your child will lose interest in nursing at a particular age. Some authorities report that this occurs at nine or ten months; others pinpoint the one-year mark. There are further conflicting claims that babies are likely to initiate weaning anytime between eighteen months and four years.

Many women we met, however, reported that their babies never showed any signs of losing interest in nursing. The concept that there exists a magic window of opportunity when weaning is especially easy can be misleading and unfortunate. If your child *does* indicate reduced interest in nursing, that can certainly make your job of weaning easier. If, on the other hand, you don't observe this phenomenon, it doesn't mean that you missed it or that your baby has failed to go through some normal stage. It simply means that you might have to decide to wean without the benefit of a clear signal from your baby.

• Think about whether you plan to wean to a bottle or cup. This decision will depend on both your child's need to suck and his ability to get sufficient liquids using only a cup. If you look to the experts for advice, you will find a wide range of recommendations. Some suggest weaning to a cup after your baby is seven months old so that you will not have to wean him from the bottle later. Others say that a child has strong sucking needs until he is two years old and therefore needs a bottle until then. Once again, in your role as mother, you will have to judge which is best for your child.

• If you plan to substitute a bottle, it can be useful to offer one (perhaps containing breastmilk) to your baby occasionally before you seriously begin weaning.

• Find one or two allies you can depend on for support while weaning. You will probably need as much support during this period as you did when you began nursing. One mother, who weaned her son when he was thirteen months old, said, "My friend told me, 'Anytime it gets rough and you just can't take it—bring Jason over here and I'll take good care of him.' I never had to," the mother reported, "but I thought of that so many times."

Perhaps the best way to approach this process is to realize that your decision to begin weaning is not irrevocable. You cannot predict whether your choice will be the best one until you try it. Once you try, you can watch your baby's and your own reactions, then decide whether you want to continue or not. You can begin weaning, then stop if you or your baby are not ready after all. You can cut down to a couple of favorite nursings a day, then continue these as long as you wish.

Weaning is not a demonstration of who is in control. You do not have to worry about spoiling your child if you decide, on the basis of his behavior, that he is not ready to stop nursing yet. Your job is to keep both of your best interests in mind, not to prove who is boss.

The Process of Weaning

As mentioned earlier, weaning can take weeks or months to complete. Yet its ultimate goal is to bring nursing to a close. Each mother-baby partnership must find the style and pace most suitable for itself.

One method of weaning has been suggested by La Leche League for mothers who wish to wean as their children lose interest in nursing. La Leche League suggests that mothers who think their children are ready to wean stop offering their breast for nursing. Breastfeed only when your child asks, but never refuse your child's request to nurse. Over time, your child's requests will become less frequent, and eventually they will stop.

Another way of weaning includes finding good substitutes for nursing and watching your child's reactions. Thinking of finding good substitutes is more useful than thinking of dropping or eliminating feedings because it focuses on what you're going to do while you're not nursing. For an infant of about seven months or younger, being held and cuddled while being fed from a bottle may be a good substitute. For an older child, sitting down with (and physically close to) mommy for a snack or cuddling for a story may be best.

These two styles of weaning are not completely different in practice. Both involve doing something besides nursing at times when you used to nurse. Both involve watching the child for cues as to which nursings will be easiest to replace. Both involve providing love and affection in other tangible ways as the amount of nursing time gets smaller.

In its simplest form, weaning by substitution means systematically providing a good substitute for one feeding at a time until you are no longer nursing. Within about three to seven days your body will stop producing milk at that time, and your baby should be easy to engage in other activities. If you are actively weaning, you may then decide on the next feeding for which to provide a substitute. Continue with this pattern until your baby is completely weaned. If you were nursing five times a day before you began, you may have totally weaned within three to five weeks. In some cases, especially with young babies who are accustomed to bottles, the process of weaning does proceed just that smoothly. In many instances, however, the course of weaning is much less predictable.

Mothers who have been asked how weaning is going often reply, "It depends on the day you ask." In real life, babies get sick or don't like substitutes, mothers get busy, unexpected trips come up, and textbook weaning flies out the window. So, expect difficulties and take heart in the fact that many mothers who have weaned their children report that their progress seemed to be a series of two steps forward and three steps back. For example, one mother said, "I thought my fifteen-month-old was almost weaned—we were down to one feeding a day. Then she got an ear infection that wouldn't clear up, and it seemed that nursing was a comfort to her. I also thought that it might help to fight the infection, so we were back to nursing almost continuously for a month."

Another reported, "My fourteen-month-old was nursing just once or twice a day—bedtime and sometimes at naptime. Then he and I went to visit my mother, where he slept in a port-a-crib. He couldn't sleep. He kept bumping into the sides, so I took him into bed with me. He nursed all night. I was worried we'd have to start weaning all over. But once we got home and he was in his own bed, we were back to nursing just once or twice a day."

A third mother commented, "I really tried to cut down the number of times I nursed my one-year-old, but he would not cooperate. One day I'd keep us busy, shopping, going to playgrounds, and being out all day. He'd nurse one time, but the next day he wouldn't want to leave my breast."

Despite these apparent difficulties and setbacks, all three of these mothers have weaned their children. Their flexibility in responding to these unpredicted events ultimately made weaning a more gentle and satisfying experience. These mothers and others whom we interviewed repeatedly mentioned the following four guidelines as helpful in both finding good substitutes for nursing and encouraging their children to accept them.

1. Give your child extra affection while weaning. You don't want to eliminate the warmth and comfort that are part of nursing; you just want to attach the affection to other activities. Some mothers find that their children enjoy being rocked while reading a story as much as being rocked while nursing. One mother found that she had more success when she held her child in a nonnursing position during story time.

2. Change your routines associated with nursing. Some mothers find weaning is easiest in the summer when outdoor activities can be used to the hilt—walks, picnics, playgrounds, and pools can be attractive substitutes for nursing. But remember, children are especially thirsty in the summer. Offer many substitutes to drink.

The main routine mothers struggle to change is bedtime because, in many families, everyone is accustomed to the child being nursed to sleep. Mothers reported managing this transition in a number of ways. Some told of leaving the house at night and letting the father take over putting the child to bed. One mother began to read the same book each night while rocking her baby. She would then put him into his crib, read the story one more time, and then pat him as he fell asleep. She said this routine took about twenty-five minutes and lasted about one month. After that, her son was content to be put in his crib right away and have his back rubbed without a story.

Changing routines is not always convenient or easy. The new bedtime practices often take much longer than the former nursing ones. Going to sleep is a major transition in a child's day. Many children need help in calming themselves and settling down to rest. Once nursing is part of that calming process, it usually works very efficiently. The child is conditioned to relax while nursing. Remov-

ing the rhythmic, warm, and satisfying sensations of nursing from
this transition time makes falling asleep much more difficult for the
child who has grown accustomed to them.

Weaning is the time when your young child begins to learn
other ways of going to sleep. He will need your help as he develops
his own style. Your job is to provide the consistent affectionate
framework—the story, the rocking, the song, the patting—within
which he can begin to quiet himself. In time he will learn to
quiet himself with increasing ease, and your role in the routine will
diminish.

3. If you are nursing an older infant or toddler, talk to him
about weaning. One mother said she and Jamie, her twenty-month-
old son, talked about babies a lot while weaning. They talked about
what Jamie could do that babies couldn't do. This dialogue became
part of Jamie's ritual before falling asleep. His mother said talking
was good for her, too. It soothed her and reminded her of the things
she and Jamie could still do together.

Another mother described how she used talking to help end the
process of weaning her twenty-three-month-old daughter. They had
begun weaning about four months earlier, when Debby was nursing
about four times a day. Finally, the mother felt it was time to find
a substitute for their last remaining nursing, which occurred at bedtime. So as she rocked and nursed Debby, she would say, "Mommy's
milk is going away. One day it will be all gone." She said this every
night for about two weeks. Then, on January 6—two years later this
mother remembered the date!—when Debby asked to nurse, her
mother said, "There's no more milk. Can I sing to you instead?"
Debby said, "Okay," thus beginning their new rocking and singing
routine.

4. For your older infant or child, use rules about when and
where nursing can take place. To reduce the number of nursing
times, mothers reported using phrases such as "This is juice time, not
nursing time," "We can only nurse in the rocking chair," and "Let's
save up mommy's milk for bedtime."

One mother who called herself a "closet nurser" had a twenty-two-month-old who had nursed during the night for the preceding year. She described how he had been weaned on a trip. They were at her brother's graduation and planned to stay in a hotel for four days. "The first evening there, I said, 'John, we don't nurse in a hotel.' For some reason he accepted it and did not ask. He did ask to nurse a few times after we left, but he was easily dissuaded after the four-day break."

Life after Weaning

Women who reported satisfaction with their nursing experience and who had psychologically weaned before physically weaning had the most positive feelings about ending the nursing relationship. Women who had felt compelled to wean for reasons beyond their control, such as medical problems or the need to return to work or pressure from others, often described a lingering ambivalence about whether they had made the right decision. Regardless of the reason for or readiness to wean, however, many women experienced the blues or sadness for a short time as they realized their babies were growing up. One mother compared her feelings to those she had when she packed away her child's baby clothes—a nostalgia for what had passed and would never be again.

On the other hand, several mothers reported feeling much better than they had expected once nursing was ended. The process of weaning also prepared them for its completion. One mother said she wanted to enjoy the last time she nursed her daughter. She tried to get herself into a sentimental mood so she would always remember this special final occasion. But she couldn't do it. She felt relaxed, was distracted as they nursed, and finished without any emotional fanfare.

Physically, mothers reported different reactions to weaning. Some women reported having painfully full breasts for two to seven days whereas others felt no discomfort at all. Some mothers lost several pounds without trying, and others had to reduce their calorie

intake substantially to avoid gaining weight. Some described themselves as feeling more attractive after weaning; others reported no
change. Likewise, some reported sex getting noticeably better, and
others experienced no change in sex. Many mothers, however, reported feeling less tired and more energetic once breastfeeding was
completed.

Some mothers reported mood changes following nursing, especially increased irritability, impatience, and dissatisfaction. These are
partially the result of hormonal changes accompanying the cessation
of lactation. Prolactin, a hormone related to milk production, is
associated with feelings of well-being and complacency. Thus prolactin withdrawal is likely to affect these feelings. These effects are most
noticeable with early weaning because prolactin levels are highest in
the early postpartum period.

Many mothers did not notice any major changes in their children's temperament once they were weaned. The four-month-old
who woke up every night continued to wake up; the clingy ten-
month-old stayed clingy; the cuddly nineteen-month-old still loved
to cuddle. Some mothers did, however, notice differences in their
children's eating or sleeping patterns. A few babies showed reactions
to formula. Some babies or toddlers became firmly attached to their
pacifiers or bottles. Others seemed to show spurts of independence,
especially in their willingness to move away from mother toward
fathers or siblings. It's possible, however, that certain changes would
have occurred even without weaning.

Weaning is likely to be one of your first major experiences in
letting go of your child. One mother, Marie-Bernice Downey, expressed her feelings about weaning within the wider context of
parenthood:

> I have older children who haven't been nursed for a long time; my
> "baby" is twelve years old. Parenting doesn't stop with weaning. As
> a matter of fact, the word "wean" means so much more in our modern
> language than the cessation of breastfeeding. I thought of this as I set
> the table tonight with one less dish than last night. Our college boy
> went back to school after a weekend at home. The feeling I had was

much like the twinge I felt at the weaning of my nursling. Next fall, another plate will be gone, another twinge. But this is what we raised them for, to become independent and move on. Really, there are many steps to weaning. Some of these steps are going to school, staying away overnight (camping, a p.j. party), getting a job, going to high school and college. Each is a step away, and each requires a letting go. Yes, I'm still weaning and still nurturing too, for they come back, call, and write. Even though I take a plate off, I also put it back from time to time. I hope I always will (Downey, p. 5).

Whenever the time for weaning arrives, rest assured that your nursing experience has probably taught you some important things about yourself and your baby. You have learned that you can care for another human being and can put someone else's needs before your own. You can enjoy giving. And you have learned to trust your instincts—to have confidence that you know this child and can usually interpret and satisfy his needs. You have also learned to trust him. You can rely on him to know when he is hungry and when he has had enough, to know when he is ready to explore and when he needs to touch base.

Much of this understanding probably has come from your hundreds of interactions each day, many of which had nothing to do with nursing. But much also must have emerged from your nursing experience. Since breastfeeding cannot be carried on according to immutable guidelines from some outside source, you have grown in your role as a mother who has had to make judgments over and over again regarding your baby's needs and preferences. Breastfeeding is unique in that it unites a mother and baby in a synchronized and reciprocal physical relationship. It has offered you intimate opportunities to become attuned to each other and has helped you to establish a rhythm and pattern of parenting. It is likely that the legacies of your breastfeeding experience will continue to shape your relationship with each other.

References

American Academy of Pediatrics. "Breastfeeding." *Pediatrics* 62 (1979): 591–601.

———. "The Promotion of Breast-feeding." *Pediatrics* 69 (1982): 654–61.

———, Committee on Nutrition. "Encouraging Breast-feeding." *Pediatrics* 65 (1980): 657.

Barber, V., and Skaggs, M. M. *The Mother Person.* New York: Bobbs-Merrill, 1975.

Barnes, G. R., Lethin, A. N., Jr., Jackson, E. B., and Shea, N. "Management of Breast-feeding." *Journal of the American Medical Association* 151 (1953): 192–97.

Ben Shaul, D. M. "The Composition of the Milk of Wild Animals." *The International Zoo Year Book.* Vol. 4. Edited by Carolyn Jarvis and D. Morris. London: Hutchinson, 1962.

Brazelton, T. B. "Behavioral Competence of the Newborn Infant." *Seminars in Perinatology* 3 (1979): 35–44.

Brazelton, T. B., Koslowski, B., and Main, M. In M. Lewis and L. A. Rosenblum, eds., *The Effect of the Infant on Its Caregiver.* New York: John Wiley & Sons, 1974.

Brewster, D. P. *You Can Breastfeed Your Baby—Even in Special Situations.* Emmaus, Pa.: Rodale Press, 1979.

De Carvalho, M., Robertson, S., Merkatz, R., and Klaus, M. H. "Milk Intake and Frequency of Feeding in Breast-fed Infants." *Early Human Development* 7 (1983).

Downey, Marie-Bernice. *Virginia Visions.* Special Edition, 1980.

Fantz, R. L. "The Origin of Form Perception." *Scientific American* 204 (1961): 66–72.

Frantz, K. B., and Kalmen, B. A. "Breastfeeding Works for Cesareans, Too." *R.N.* 42 (1979): 39–47.

Goldfarb, J., and Tibbetts, E. *Breastfeeding Handbook: A Practical Reference for Physicians, Nurses, and Other Professionals.* Hillside, N.J.: Enslow Publishers, 1980.

Grad, R., Bush, D., Guyer, R., Acevedo, Z., Trause, M. A., and Reukauf, D. *The Father Book: Pregnancy and Beyond.* Washington, D.C.: Acropolis Books, 1981.

Guyer, R. L., and Freivogel, M. W. *Why Breastfeed?* Alexandria, Va.: Alliance for Perinatal Research and Services, 1981.

Health Education Associates. Pamphlets on Breastfeeding. Glenside, Pa.: Health Education Associates, Inc.

Jelliffe, D. B., and Jelliffe, E. F. P. *Human Milk in the Modern World.* Oxford: Oxford University Press, 1978.

Kitzinger, S. *The Experience of Breastfeeding.* New York: Penguin Books, 1980.

———. *Women as Mothers: How They See Themselves in Different Cultures.* New York: Random House, 1978.

Klaus, M. H., and Kennell, J. H. *Maternal-Infant Bonding.* St. Louis: C. V. Mosby Co., 1976.

———. *Parent-Infant Bonding.* 2d ed. St. Louis: C. V. Mosby Co., 1982.

La Leche League International. *The Womanly Art of Breastfeeding.* 3d ed. Franklin Park, Ill.: La Leche League International, 1981.

Lawrence, R. A. *Breast-feeding: A Guide for the Medical Profession.* St. Louis: C. V. Mosby Co., 1980.

Lozoff, Betsy. "The Sensitive Period: An Anthropological View." Paper presented at the meetings of the Society for Research in Child Development, New Orleans, 1977.

Lozoff, B., and Brittenham, G. "Infant Care—Cache or Carry?" *Journal of Pediatrics* 95 (1979): 478–83.

Lucas, A., and Baum, J. D. "Differences in the Pattern of Milk Intake between Breast and Bottle Fed Infants." *Early Human Development* 5 (1981): 195–99.

Macdonald, J. "The Working Mother and Her Breastfeeding Infant." *Canadian Nurse,* March 1983, pp. 21–23.

Macfarlane, A. *The Psychology of Childbirth.* Cambridge, Mass.: Harvard University Press, 1977.

Martinez, G. A., and Nalezienski, J. P. "The Recent Trend in Breast-feeding." *Pediatrics* 64 (1979): 686–92.

Masters, W. H., and Johnson, V. E. *Human Sexual Response.* Boston: Little, Brown, 1966.

Meara, H. "La Leche League in the United States: A Key to Successful Breast-feeding in Non-supportive Culture." *Journal of Nurse-Midwifery* 21 (1976): 20–26.

Newton, N. "Psychological Differences between Breast and Bottle Feeding." *American Journal of Clinical Nutrition* 24 (1971): 993–1004.

Newton, N., and Newton, M. "Mothers' Reactions to Their Newborn Babies." *Journal of the American Medical Association* 181 (1962): 206–11.

————. "Psychological Aspects of Lactation." *New England Journal of Medicine* 277 (1967): 1179–87.

Oakley, A. *Becoming a Mother.* New York: Schocken Books, 1979.

Raphael, D. *The Tender Gift: Breastfeeding.* New York: Schocken Books, 1973.

Riordan, J. *A Practical Guide to Breastfeeding.* St. Louis: C. V. Mosby Co., 1983.

Scott, JoAnne. Personal communication.

Sears, W. *Nighttime Parenting: How to Get Your Baby and Child to Sleep.* Franklin Park, Ill.: La Leche League International, 1985.

Stein, S. B. *The New Baby.* New York: Walker & Co., 1974.

Stewart, D., and Gaiser, C. "Supporting Lactation When Mothers and Infants Are Separated: A Clinical Guideline for Perinatal Nurses." *Nursing Clinics of North America* 13 (1978): 47–61.

Van Esterik, P., and Greiner, T. "Breastfeeding and Women's Work: Constraints and Opportunities." *Studies in Family Planning* 12 (1981): 184–97.

Waletzky, L. "Husband's Problems with Breastfeeding." *American Journal of Orthopsychiatry* 49 (1979): 349–52.

Winnicott, Donald W. *The Family and Individual Development.* London: Tavistock Publications, 1978.

Index

Diane M. Reukauf is an ASPO-certified childbirth educator. She has a master's degree in counseling and is pursuing doctoral studies at the University of Virginia. She is currently teaching courses in psychology and human development at Northern Virginia Community College, and lectures widely to hospital and medical groups on the subject of the post-partum period and sexuality. She is co-author of *The Father Book* and lives in Alexandria, Virginia, with her husband and three children.

Mary Anne Trause received her Ph.D. in human development from Cornell University and is currently in her fourth year of postdoctoral work in clinical psychology at the University of Virginia. She has done extensive research on the newborn in intensive care units, and is currently working at the Family Counseling Center in Dale City, Virginia. She is co-author of *The Father Book* and lives in Alexandria, Virginia, with her husband and two children.